Cardiology Explained

Cardiology Explained

W. M. Drake
Department of Medicine,
St Bartholomew's Hospital, London

P. A. Broadhurst
Department of Cardiology,
St Bartholomew's Hospital, London

D. S. Dymond
Department of Cardiology,
St Bartholomew's Hospital, London

CHAPMAN & HALL MEDICAL

London · Weinheim · New York · Tokyo · Melbourne · Madras

Published by Chapman & Hall, 2–6 Boundary Row, London SE1 8HN, UK

Chapman & Hall, 2–6 Boundary Row, London SE1 8HN, UK

Chapman & Hall GmbH, Pappelallee 3, 69469 Weinheim, Germany

Chapman & Hall USA, 115 Fifth Avenue, New York, NY 10003, USA

Chapman & Hall Japan, ITP-Japan, Kyowa Building, 3F, 2–2–1 Hirakawacho, Chiyoda-ku, Tokyo 102, Japan

Chapman & Hall Australia, 102 Dodds Street, South Melbourne, Victoria 3205, Australia

Chapman & Hall India, R. Seshadri, 32 Second Main Road, CIT East, Madras 600 035, India

First edition 1997

© 1997 W. M. Drake, P. A. Broadhurst, D. S. Dymond

Typeset in 10½/12pt Times by Type Study, Scarborough

Printed in Great Britain by Cambridge University Press

ISBN 0 412 73680 2

∞ Printed on permanent acid-free text paper, manufactured in accordance with ANSI/NISO Z39.48–1992 and ANSI/NISO Z39.48–1984 (Permanence of Paper).

Contents

Preface

Cardiology is a subject that is often poorly understood and consequently feared by many students and junior doctors. Auscultatory findings are new and can be bewildering and the investigations, such as the ECG are perceived as difficult to master. Yet the subject is centred around physiological and pharmacological principles with which all students and doctors are familiar from an early stage in their training. Our aim in writing this book has been to provide a text that recaps those principles and uses them to explain, in clear language, the common cardiovascular diseases, their presentation, diagnosis, and treatment. Where additional background information is required, this is presented in tinted boxes so as not to interrupt the logical flow of the text. There are also sample case histories to illustrate certain points and help commit them to memory, as well as several summary boxes. Although by no means an exhaustive text, *Cardiology Explained* contains all the factual information needed for medical finals and will therefore be useful for students as well as General Practitioners and junior Hospital doctors. We hope that the easy-to-read style of the text will remove the fear and mystique of the subject and instil confidence and enthusiasm in the reader.

WMD
PAB
DSD

Principal author's note

Although there are three authors on the cover of this text there is a fourth person who has read every word several times over and provided limitless enthusiasm and encouragement during its preparation. Her name is Melanie Hiorns, she is shortly to be my wife and it is to her that I dedicate my share of the book.

WMD

Acknowledgements

We would like to express our gratitude to Dr Janet Dacie, Dr Simon Rees, Professor Keith Britton and Dr Sanjay Sharma for their kindness in providing X-ray material for inclusion in the book. Also to Dr Se Cullen for his help with the chapter on congenital heart disease. Thanks also go to Dr Julian Allwood for the generous loan of his computer, to Rocky Broadhurst for his constant inspiration and to Dr Alistair Chesser for his incalculable contribution.

WMD
PAB
DSD

History and examination $\boxed{1}$

HISTORY TAKING

The history and physical examination play an essential role in the diagnosis and management of a patient with suspected cardiovascular disease. This chapter will deal with cardiac symptoms and describe the techniques used in making a clinical assessment of the cardiovascular system.

Chest pain

A carefully taken history with particular attention to the quality of the pain, its radiation and relationship to certain precipitating and relieving factors is needed in order to differentiate the many causes of chest pain. Pain due to **myocardial ischaemia** is called **angina pectoris** and occurs when there is an imbalance between myocardial oxygen demand and supply. The severity of the symptoms is variable and not all patients perceive angina as pain. Most patients describe a 'constricting', 'choking' sensation or a tightness or heaviness across the anterior chest wall. Pain fibres from the heart enter the cervical spinal cord at the same level as fibres from the arms, neck and jaw so it is not infrequent for pain to radiate to or be felt in one or more of these sites. Most attacks of angina are precipitated by physical or emotional stress and are relieved within a few minutes by rest. Another characteristic feature is that the pain of angina is usually relieved by **sublingual nitrates** and where there is diagnostic doubt this is often helpful. Many patients dismiss the symptoms of angina as being due to 'indigestion'.

The pain of **myocardial infarction** is usually of similar quality to that of angina but is characteristically more intense, lasts longer and is not relieved by rest or sublingual nitrates. Pain due to inflammation of the pericardium (**pericarditis**) often has a sharp stabbing quality made worse by respiration and relieved by sitting forward. **Dissection of the aorta** classically causes a sudden intense chest pain, often radiating to an area on the back between the shoulder blades. It may be difficult to distinguish from the pain of myocardial infarction.

Dyspnoea

This is a common cardiac symptom and is the subjective sensation of breathlessness. Normal people feel breathless during vigorous exercise but in cardiac disease it occurs inappropriately to the degree of physical activity. Clinically it is helpful to establish a patient's functional capability by asking how far they can walk or how many stairs they can climb before pausing for breath. Exertional dyspnoea is most commonly associated with heart failure and the mechanisms are discussed in that chapter. **Orthopnoea** refers to the sensation of breathlessness when lying flat and is relieved when an upright posture is adopted. **Paroxysmal nocturnal dyspnoea (PND)** is the symptom of waking at night fighting for breath, often associated with sweating. Sitting up or getting out of bed often relieves the symptoms. Patients with orthopnoea and PND frequently sleep propped up at night.

Palpitations

This is an awareness of the heart beating and may be a normal phenomenon or occur as a symptom of serious cardiac pathology. Anxiety and exercise are common causes of palpitation that are not due to serious heart disease. Patients may describe the feeling of their hearts having 'missed a beat' but in fact this represents the compensatory pause that follows an extrasystole. Palpitations due to paroxysmal tachycardia tend to start and finish abruptly. Ventricular and supraventricular tachycardias are generally felt by the patient to be regular in rhythm, whereas atrial fibrillation may cause the sensation of an irregular heartbeat.

Dizziness and syncope

Sudden falls in blood pressure reduce cerebral perfusion. Brain tissue is exquisitely sensitive to metabolic changes so that loss of consciousness usually follows within 10 seconds of the cessation of cerebral blood flow. This is called **syncope**. When patients feel dizzy and as though they are about to lose consciousness, the term **pre-syncope** is used. Syncopal attacks are characterized by hypotension and pallor, followed by loss of consciousness. Recovery is rapid, usually within a minute, if the underlying problem is rectified. Cardiac disorders that may result in syncope and pre-syncope include disturbances of rhythm (either tachycardias or bradycardias) or obstructions to cardiac output such as a narrowed (stenosed) aortic valve. Another common cause is **postural hypotension**. With age or with conditions that damage the autonomic nerve supply, such as diabetes, there may be impaired function of the baroreceptor mediated reflexes that control blood pressure. As the patient stands up there is reduced or delayed reflex vasoconstriction, so blood pressure falls and pre-syncope or syncope may follow.

Ankle swelling (oedema)   cankles

Heart failure is accompanied by salt and water retention. This tends to gravitate to the feet and ankles of patients who are mobile and to the sacrum in those who are confined to bed. In cases of severe heart failure oedema may extend all the way up the leg and even produce scrotal swelling in men. Some cardiac drugs, most notably **nifedipine** and other calcium antagonists, may also cause ankle oedema.

Non-specific symptoms

Fatigue is common in heart failure and is probably due to a chronic state of underperfusion of the tissues. This symptom is also prominent in endocarditis and may occur with the use of ß-blockers for angina or hypertension. Flu-like symptoms may precede the development of pericarditis or myocarditis.

EXAMINATION OF THE CARDIOVASCULAR SYSTEM

General examination

Cardiovascular disorders, like diseases of other organs, may have systemic effects. Examination starts with general observations about the patient's overall health. **Fever** is common with heart valve infections and following myocardial infarction. Sympathetic activation due to chest pain or hypotension may cause **sweating**. Longstanding heart failure with chronic ill health may cause weight loss and, in severe cases, **cachexia**. Poor tissue oxygenation may cause peripheral and/or central **cyanosis**. **Oedema** is common in patients with heart failure. Sustained gentle pressure over the ankle or the anterior border of the tibia produces an indentation in the contour of the skin in patients with dependent oedema.

Clubbing (Fig. 1.1) refers to a spongy enlargement of the tissue around the nail beds of the fingers and toes. The skin becomes shiny and

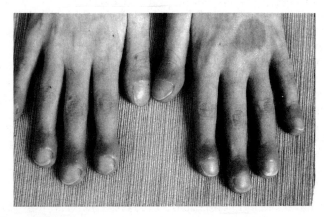

Fig. 1.1   Finger clubbing.

darker than normal and the angle between the base of the nail and the skin is lost. In the context of cardiovascular disease it is most frequently seen with **congenital lesions** where there is central cyanosis and is also rarely seen in **endocarditis**. **Splinter haemorrhages** are non-tender lesions that sometimes appear under the nails with infective endocarditis. They are non-specific; other causes for their appearance being trauma and vasculitis. Where they appear in endocarditis they are believed to be due to the deposition of immune complexes in the capillaries under the nail bed. A similar immune process in the kidney causes a **glomerulonephritis** with **microscopic haematuria**.

Pulses

With each contraction the left ventricle ejects a volume of blood into the aorta. The walls of this vessel are stretched and a pressure wave moves rapidly along the peripheral arteries where it may be palpated as the **arterial pulse**. It is important to palpate all of the peripheral pulses when assessing the cardiovascular system, but the radial and carotid pulses provide most information.

The **radial pulse** is palpated by gentle pressure of the artery against the distal shaft of the radius. It provides information about rate and rhythm although significant abnormalities in character may be detected. Rate is given as so many beats per minute. If the pulse is regular it is safe to count the number of beats in 15 seconds and multiply by 4. An irregular pulse requires palpation for a full minute.

A pulse is said to be **regular** if the examiner can predict when the next beat will arrive. **Irregular** pulses may either be totally **chaotic** (usually due to **atrial fibrillation**) or have an underlying regular rhythm with extra beats (**extrasystoles**) or pauses (**dropped beats**). If a pulse is totally irregular the rate is better assessed by auscultation at the apex.

Pulse character is best assessed by gentle palpation of the **carotid artery** against the transverse processes of the cervical vertebrae. A normal waveform of the carotid pulse is shown in Fig. 1.2. Left ventricular output creates the **upstroke** of the pulse. Towards the end of systole pressure in the aorta falls off but a further rapid fall like that seen in the left ventricle is prevented by closure of the aortic valve. This is called the **dicrotic notch** and is not detectable clinically. After the dicrotic notch there follows a more gentle decline in aortic pressure as blood runs off into the peripheral circulation. It is not possible to detect slight variations from the normal character of the pulse but in certain conditions of aortic valve dysfunction abnormalities of pulse waveform may be felt that reflect the underlying haemodynamic disturbances. The most important of these are **slow rising** and **collapsing** pulses.

'Slow rising' or plateau pulse

If the outlet of the left ventricle becomes narrowed (stenosed) then the carotid upstroke rises more slowly and is prolonged as the ventricle

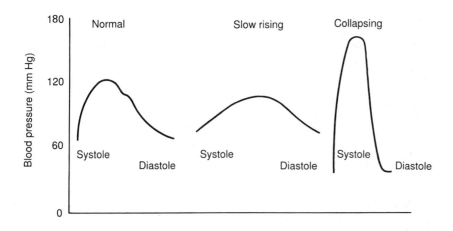

Fig. 1.2 Contrasting waveforms of normal, slow rising and collapsing arterial pulses.

requires more time to complete its emptying across the stenosed valve. This is called a plateau or slow rising pulse and its contour is compared to a normal pulse in Fig. 1.2.

Large volume or 'collapsing' pulses

The character of the downstroke depends partly on how quickly blood runs off into the circulation and partly on whether the aortic valve is able to prevent reflux of blood back into the left ventricle and maintain diastolic blood pressure. In conditions where peripheral resistance is very low (such as sepsis where toxins cause vasodilatation) blood flows unimpeded into the peripheral circulation and the carotid downstroke is abrupt. A similar pulse is felt in aortic regurgitation where blood flows back into the left ventricle during diastole and diastolic pressure is low. In both of these conditions the left ventricle contracts forcefully during *Starling* systole in order to maintain a satisfactory mean blood pressure. A pulse contour is created in which the upstroke and downstroke are steep, as shown in Fig. 1.2. This is called a **collapsing pulse** and is often best appreciated in the radial pulse. With the examiner's fingers wrapped around the patient's wrist and held in the air the pulse seems to slap against the palpating fingers.

   The volume of the peripheral pulse is dictated not only by the function of the aortic valve but also by the state of vasodilatation of the peripheral circulation. Small volume 'thready' pulses are characteristic of states such as severe haemorrhage in which there is intense vasoconstriction in order to maintain blood pressure. Large volume, bounding and even 'collapsing' pulses are felt with hyperdynamic, vasodilated states such as **fever** and **thyrotoxicosis**.

Blood pressure

Blood pressure may be measured with the use of a stethoscope and an inflatable cuff connected to an instrument called a **sphygmomanometer**. This technique relies on the principle that when pressure on a compressed artery is gradually released blood flow through the partially occluded artery is turbulent. This turbulence may be auscultated over an artery (most conveniently the brachial artery) and the points at which the sounds change in intensity correlate with systemic arterial pressures.

Accurate assessment of the blood pressure using the sphygmomanometer requires careful technique. Patients should be allowed an adequate period of relaxation before taking the blood pressure. They may sit or lie on a couch but the level of the cuff should be at the level of the heart. The correct sized cuff should be used as a small cuff on a large arm will give falsely high readings. If the circumference of the arm is more than 35 cm a large cuff is required. After inflating the cuff to 20 mmHg beyond the point at which the radial pulse disappears the cuff should be deflated at a rate of 2–3 mm/s with the column of mercury at eye level. Both systolic and diastolic values are recorded. The difference between these two values is called the pulse pressure. Certain conditions of the aortic valve may cause important abnormalities of pulse pressure and these are discussed in Chapter 5 (valvular heart disease).

Korotkoff sounds

The relationship to the sounds heard over a partially occluded vessel to direct measurements of arterial pressure were first recorded by **Korotkoff**, a Russian physician. When the pressure in a cuff applied around the upper arm exceeds systolic blood pressure there is no flow down the artery and no noise is heard over the brachial artery. As the cuff is deflated flow resumes when systolic pressure is just able to overcome pressure in the cuff. Flow is limited and turbulent and this may be auscultated with a stethoscope placed over the brachial artery. The point at which flow first becomes audible is the **first Korotkoff sound** and correlates with systolic blood pressure. As pressure is lowered further there occur subtle changes in the pitch and volume of the noises heard over the artery. These are the **second and third Korotkoff sounds** and are not important clinically. With further lowering of the pressure in the cuff the artery becomes less compressed. Flow becomes less turbulent and the sounds over the brachial artery become muffled. This is the **fourth Korotkoff sound**. Shortly after this the sounds die away completely as flow is unimpeded by the cuff. This is the **fifth Korotkoff sound** and is believed to correlate most accurately with direct measurements of diastolic blood pressure.

Jugular venous pulse (JVP)

There are no valves between the internal jugular veins and the right atrium (RA). Hence important information about changes in right atrial pressure during the cardiac cycle may be inferred from examination of the jugular veins and their pulsations. Two main observations are made. First, the height of the JVP above a fixed anatomical landmark (generally the sternal angle) is used as a measure of right atrial pressure. The sternal angle is roughly 5 cm above the right atrium, so that a JVP visible 4 cm above the sternal angle corresponds to a central venous pressure of 9 cm water. Second, the waveform of the JVP gives more detailed diagnostic information, although this is difficult and requires practise. The oscillations of the JVP usually comprise two elevations and two troughs (Fig. 1.3). The first elevation (the **'a' wave**) is caused by a rise in right atrial pressure due to atrial contraction. This is followed by right ventricular contraction which pulls the tricuspid valve down. Combined with atrial relaxation, this causes a fall in right atrial pressure, producing the **'x' descent**. As right ventricular contraction continues, venous return into a closed RA causes the second elevation, the **'v' wave**. At the end of ventricular contraction the tricuspid valve opens. Blood flows passively into the right ventricle so pressure in the right atrium falls, producing the **'y' descent**. The 'a' wave is the most convenient oscillation to identify and occurs fractionally before the onset of ventricular systole, which can be timed by palpation of the carotid pulse.

For inspection of the JVP, patients should be positioned with the upper body at 45° to the bed and with the neck held in slight flexion by a pillow to relax the sternomastoid muscles (see Fig. 1.4). It should be

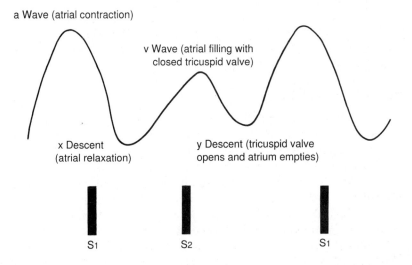

Fig. 1.3 Waveform of the normal jugular venous pulse. (For explanation of heart sounds see p. 10.)

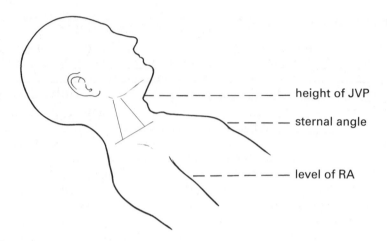

— height of JVP

— sternal angle

— level of RA

Fig. 1.4 Positioning of the patient for assessment of the jugular venous pulse.

possible to see the pulsations of the internal jugular vein on either side of the neck. It is important to distinguish between the double waveform of the JVP and the single, palpable pulsation arising from the carotid artery.

Abnormalities of the JVP include those of height and waveform. A JVP more than 4 cm above the sternal angle implies that RA pressures are high. This is most commonly due to right heart failure. If the venous pressure is significantly elevated it may be necessary to sit a patient up in order to identify the top of the pulsations. If the JVP cannot be seen at 45° then lowering the patient to 30° or less may reveal the pulsations. Alternatively, the **hepato-jugular reflux** may be used. Gentle pressure over the liver displaces blood from the hepatic sinusoids and leads to a transient increase in right atrial pressure. Sometimes engorged neck veins are due to superior vena cava obstruction, distinguished by the absence of any pulsation. Abnormalities of waveform are discussed in the section on Tricuspid regurgitation in Chapter 5.

Praecordial palpation

Palpation of the praecordium is used mainly to assess heart size and the presence of ventricular hypertrophy. Sometimes blood flow across a valve or between chambers is so turbulent as to be palpable. These are called **thrills**. Occasionally heart sounds (valve closures) are palpable. When the heart contracts it creates an impulse on the chest wall. The most lateral and inferior point at which this can be felt is called the **apex beat**. In normal people the apex beat is felt in the 5th intercostal space in the mid-clavicular line and is created mainly by the left ventricular impulse (Fig. 1.5).

The apex beat may be abnormal in position or character. **Displacements** of the apex may occur with movements of the whole heart (such as in tension pneumothorax where the entire mediastinum is

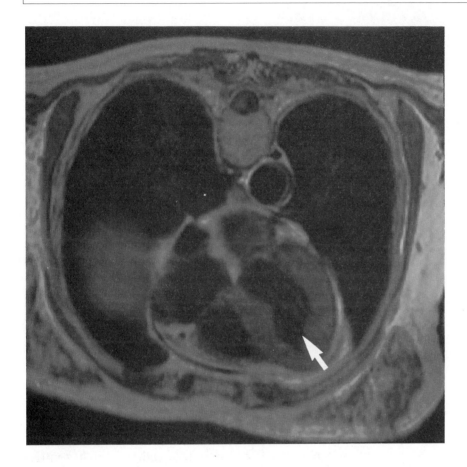

Fig. 1.5 Transverse section of the thorax (MRI scan) at the level of the 5th intercostal space. At this level, the muscle lying under the chest wall is almost exclusively left ventricle (arrow).

shifted) or if a particular chamber becomes overloaded. Any condition with an increased volume of blood present in the left ventricle at the end of diastole will cause the apex to be felt more laterally and inferiorly than normal. Conditions in which there is increased resistance to left ventricular emptying, such as a narrowed (stenosed) aortic valve or hypertension, lead to thickening (hypertrophy) of ventricular muscle. This causes a **thrusting apex beat** in which the palpating fingers become lifted off the chest wall by the force of contraction of the increased muscle mass.

The right ventricle lies under the left hand side of the sternum and the 4th and 5th rib spaces on that side (Fig. 1.6). If the right ventricle contracts very forcefully then it pushes against the inside of the chest wall. If the heel of the hand is placed to the left of the sternum over the right ventricle with the fingers pointing upwards then the hand will feel as though it is being lifted off the chest wall. This is called a **right**

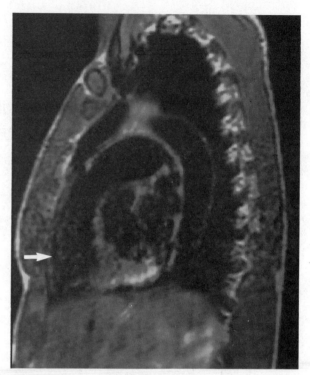

Fig. 1.6 Sagittal MR scan just to the left of the sternum. Muscle underneath the chest wall here is almost exclusively right ventricle (arrow).

ventricular lift or **parasternal heave** and suggests that the right ventricle is under strain. This is most commonly due to high pressures in the pulmonary arteries such that the right ventricle has to work harder than usual in order to drive blood through the pulmonary circulation.

Heart sounds

In order to understand heart sounds it is necessary to recap events in the cardiac cycle. During diastole, pressure in the left atrium exceeds that in the relaxed left ventricle and blood flows across the open mitral valve. At the start of ventricular systole pressure within the ventricle rapidly exceeds that in the left atrium. The mitral valve is forced shut, producing the first heart sound, S_1. As left ventricular contraction continues pressure within this chamber rises and exceeds pressure in the aorta, forcing open the aortic valve. As ventricular systole comes to an end pressure within the left ventricle falls. When pressure in the aorta exceeds that in the left ventricle the aortic valve closes, producing the second heart sound, S_2 (Fig. 1.7). The first heart sound is usually best heard between the lower left sternal edge and the apex. The second sound is usually best heard in the second interspace on the right. The **diaphragm** detects these relatively high pitched sounds better than the bell.

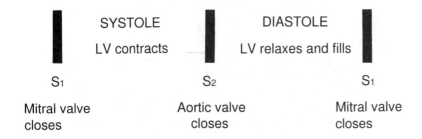

NORMAL HEART SOUNDS

SYSTOLE	DIASTOLE
LV contracts	LV relaxes and fills

S_1 S_2 S_1

Mitral valve closes Aortic valve closes Mitral valve closes

Fig. 1.7 Timing of the first and second heart sounds.

Splitting of the second heart sound

The above discussion deals only with events on the left side of the heart. Similar changes occur in the right heart involving the right atrium, right ventricle, tricuspid valve and pulmonary artery. Right ventricular and pulmonary artery pressures are lower than those in the left heart and events also occur slightly later. The second heart sound therefore has two components, termed **A_2** and **P_2**, relating to closure of the aortic and pulmonary valves respectively. With inspiration more blood is sucked into the thoracic cavity. Volumes and pressures in the right ventricular rise and this chamber prolongs its systole in order to be able to pump the extra blood into the pulmonary circulation. Closure of the pulmonary valve (P_2) occurs later and the gap between the A_2 and P_2 therefore becomes wider. With expiration right ventricular volume and output falls and the pulmonary valve closes earlier. A_2 and P_2 move closer together and may fuse to produce a single sound (Fig. 1.8). Splitting of the second heart sound can be best appreciated with the diaphragm of the stethoscope in the pulmonary area (second interspace on the left).

Added heart sounds

After closure of the aortic valve (A_2) there follows a period of rapid ventricular filling as blood flows across the mitral valve into the left ventricle (Fig. 1.9). This may be associated with an extra, low-pitched heart sound. This is a third heart sound (**S_3**) and is best heard with the bell of the stethoscope at the apex. It is not known exactly what causes S_3, but it may be due to tensing of the chordae tendinae and ventricular wall during the period of rapid filling. In children and young adults up to the age of 30, S_3 is regarded as normal, but after this age it is associated with certain pathological conditions in which the ventricle is under 'stress', such as heart failure or severe anaemia.

Passive filling during diastole is followed by a short atrial contraction, which provides an extra 'boost' to ventricular filling. Where this

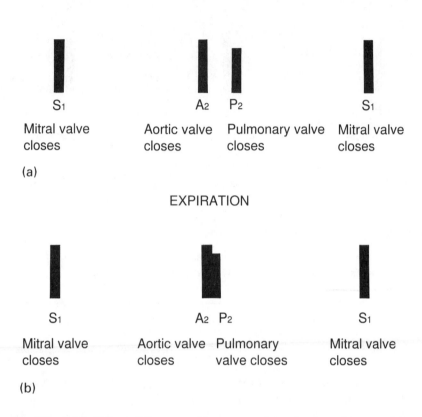

INSPIRATION

| S₁ | A₂ | P₂ | S₁ |

S₁
Mitral valve closes

A₂
Aortic valve closes

P₂
Pulmonary valve closes

S₁
Mitral valve closes

(a)

EXPIRATION

S₁
Mitral valve closes

A₂
Aortic valve closes

P₂
Pulmonary valve closes

S₁
Mitral valve closes

(b)

Fig. 1.8 (a) Splitting of the second heart sound: inspiration. Closure of the pulmonary valve is later so A₂ and P₂ separate. (b) Splitting of the second heart sound: expiration. Closure of the pulmonary valve is earlier so A₂ and P₂ move together.

THIRD HEART SOUND

S₁
Mitral valve closes

S₂
Aortic valve closes

S₃
Rapid filling early in diastole

S₁
Mitral valve closes

Fig. 1.9 Third heart sound.

contraction is abnormally powerful it may produce a low-pitched sound at the end of diastole, just before S_1 (Fig. 1.10). Again this is best heard with the bell of the stethoscope at the cardiac apex. This is a fourth heart sound (S_4) and suggests that the atrium is having to work harder than usual in order to ensure adequate diastolic filling of the left ventricle. A fourth heart sound often occurs in severe hypertension or aortic stenosis, when overworked ventricular muscle becomes very stiff and non-compliant to diastolic filling.

Gallop rhythms

The addition of either of the diastolic sounds to S_1 and S_2 creates a triple rhythm to the cardiac cycle, often referred to as a **gallop rhythm**. At fast heart rates diastole is shorter. Consequently, if both added sounds are present in a tachycardic patient they tend to merge into one, very loud extra sound. This is called a **summation gallop** (Fig. 1.11).

Heart murmurs

Heart murmurs are distinguishable from heart sounds by their longer duration and are the result of turbulent blood flow within the heart and great vessels. Murmurs may be innocent (caused by high flow across normal valves) but they may also be caused by flow across

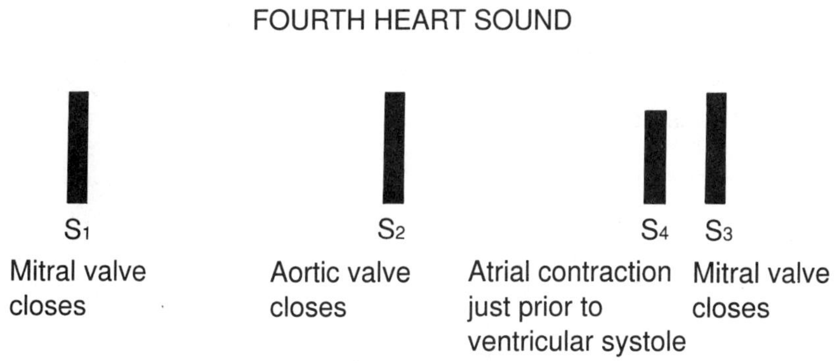

FOURTH HEART SOUND

S_1

Mitral valve closes

S_2

Aortic valve closes

S_4

Atrial contraction just prior to ventricular systole

S_3

Mitral valve closes

Fig. 1.10 Fourth heart sound.

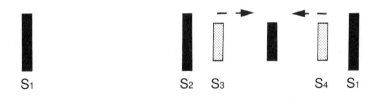

S_1

S_2 S_3

S_4 S_1

Fig. 1.11 Summation gallop. At fast heart rates diastole becomes shorter. S_3 and S_4 merge into one sound producing a summation gallop.

diseased valves or abnormal communications within the heart. A variety of characteristics are used to describe a murmur and help determine its cause. These include **location**, **radiation**, **loudness**, **quality**, and **timing**.

Location and radiation

The surface projection of the heart and its valves is shown in Fig. 1.12. The site at which a murmur is heard depends not only on the anatomical position of the valve but also on the direction of the turbulent blood flow. For example, the aortic valve is situated to the left of the sternum in the 3rd intercostal space. Blood flows out of the left ventricle through the valve into the ascending aorta along a line directed towards the 2nd intercostal space on the right and then into the carotid arteries. Consequently, systolic aortic valve murmurs are generally heard over the area outlined in Fig. 1.13 and also over the carotid vessels in the neck, although the aortic area is traditionally taken to be the second rib space to the right of the sternum. Similarly systolic mitral valve murmurs are usually heard at the cardiac apex but frequently radiate to the axilla. These and the sites where murmurs arising from other heart valves are usually heard are illustrated in Fig. 1.13.

Loudness

This is dictated by the velocity of blood flow and does not necessarily correlate with the severity of the cardiac lesion. Some people use a grading system of 1–6 but in practice it is common to use the words soft, moderately loud and loud.

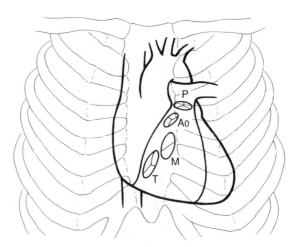

Fig. 1.12 Diagram of the surface projection of the heart and valves.
T = tricuspid; M = mitral; A0 = aortic; P = pulmonary.

Timing

Simultaneous palpation of the carotid pulse with auscultation allows murmurs to be identified as being in systole or diastole. **Systolic murmurs** occur *with* the carotid impulse whereas those in **diastole** are

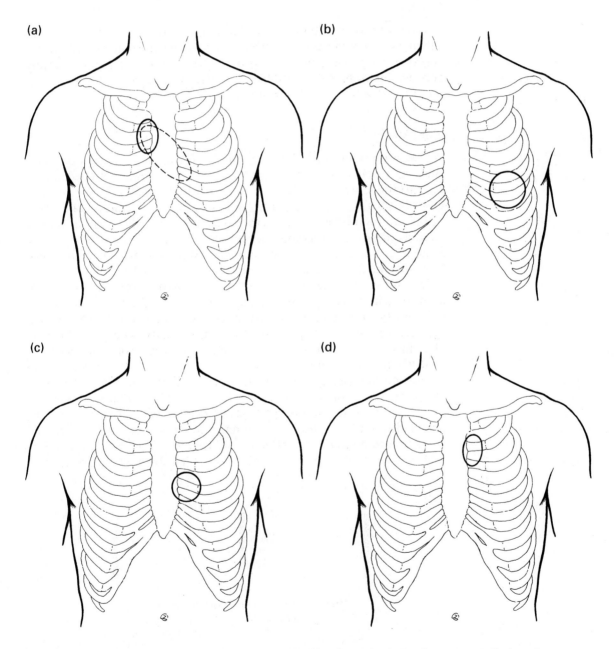

Fig. 1.13 Areas where heart sounds and murmurs arising from the four valves are usually heard. (a) aortic area, (b) mitral area, (c) tricuspid area, (d) pulmonary area.

heard *between* pulses. It is not sufficient to describe a murmur as being systolic or diastolic as different cardiac lesions may produce murmurs in the same period of the cardiac cycle but have very different characteristics. This is discussed more fully below.

Quality

A variety of terms are used to describe the noises created by different valvular defects, including 'rumbling', 'blowing', and 'harsh'. Such terms are very subjective and it is probably better to distinguish simply between high-pitched (heard best with the diaphragm) and low-pitched (heard best with the bell) murmurs.

Systolic murmurs

Where a murmur is produced by blood flowing from a high-pressure chamber (such as the ventricle) to a low-pressure chamber (such as the atrium) the murmur is said to be **pansystolic** (Fig. 1.14). This is because there is such a large pressure gradient across the leaking valve that turbulent blood flow occurs throughout ventricular systole and is unaffected by the contractile state of the ventricle as systole progresses. Systolic murmurs arising from the mitral valve are high-pitched, heard best with the diaphragm and often radiate to the axilla.

In contrast, systolic murmurs due to narrowed valves that lead out of a ventricle into a large vessel (such as narrowing of the aortic valve) vary in intensity with time. In the early stages of systole, when the ventricle is generating sufficient pressure to open the narrowed valve there is little flow and the murmur is absent. As systole progresses and the ventricle generates more pressure, flow across the valve increases and the murmur becomes louder. Towards the end of systole, as pressure in the aorta rises, flow across the valve falls off again and the murmur dies away. Such murmurs are termed **ejection systolic** (Fig. 1.15) as they are maximal in mid-systole. It is customary to draw murmurs in patients' notes according to the variation in intensity with time as shown in Figs 1.14–1.17. Systolic murmurs arising from the aortic valve are usually

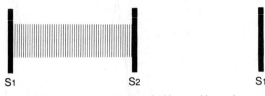

S₁   S₂   S₁

Pansystolic murmur heard with equal intensity
throughout the cardiac cycle

Fig. 1.14 Pansystolic murmurs are heard with equal intensity throughout the cardiac cycle.

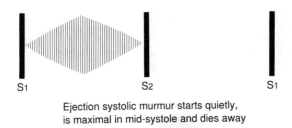

Ejection systolic murmur starts quietly,
is maximal in mid-systole and dies away

Fig. 1.15   Ejection systolic murmurs start quietly, are maximal in mid-systole and die away.

high-pitched, best heard with the diaphragm of the stethoscope and often radiate to the carotid arteries.

Diastolic murmurs

Diastolic murmurs are heard *between* carotid pulses. During normal diastole, blood flows into the ventricles across unobstructed tricuspid and mitral valves. Blood is prevented from refluxing back into the ventricles from the outflow vessels (aorta and pulmonary arteries) by the action of the aortic and pulmonary valves. It follows that diastolic murmurs may be due either to turbulent flow into the ventricles from the atria or to blood refluxing back into the ventricles from the great vessels. Again it is not sufficient to describe a murmur simply as being diastolic. If the aortic valve is incompetent then flow back into the ventricle will be maximal early in diastole when the head of pressure in the aorta favouring back flow is greatest. As diastole progresses and blood flows into the peripheral circulation, pressure in the proximal aorta declines, so blood flow back into the left ventricle falls off. The murmur of aortic regurgitation, therefore, is described as **early diastolic** (Fig. 1.16). It starts loudly and dies away, so is sometimes called a **decrescendo murmur**. The murmur of aortic regurgitation is best heard with the diaphragm of the stethoscope with the patient sitting forward in expiration.

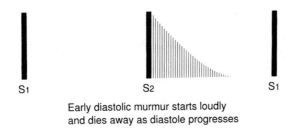

Early diastolic murmur starts loudly
and dies away as diastole progresses

Fig. 1.16   Early diastolic murmurs start loudly and die away as diastole progresses.

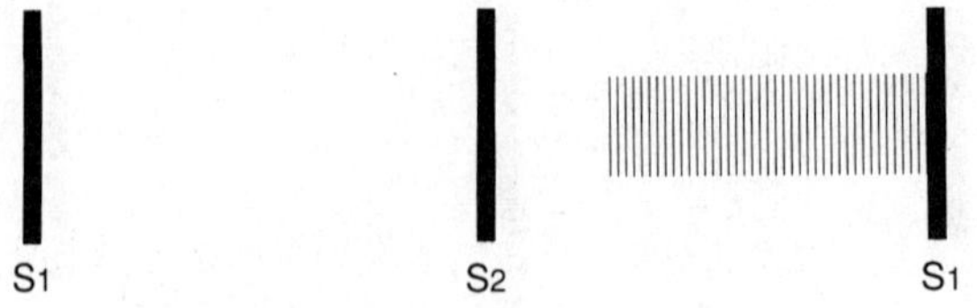

Mid-diastolic murmurs usually start
in early to mid-diastole and continue
up to the first heart sound

Fig. 1.17 Mid-diastolic murmurs usually start in early to mid-diastole and continue up to the first heart sound.

Murmurs due to turbulent flow across atrioventricular valves (such as the mitral valve) often start in early to mid-diastole and continue right up to the first sound (Fig. 1.17). In patients in sinus rhythm the murmur may become louder just prior to the first heart sound and the onset of systole. This is because atrial contraction gives an extra 'kick' to flow across the valve, increasing the turbulence and the volume of the murmur. These murmurs are usually low-pitched and rumbling and heard best with the bell of the stethoscope.

Cardiac investigations | 2

ELECTROCARDIOGRAM (ECG)

The ECG is an essential investigation in the assessment of the cardiac patient. It is a representation of the electrical changes that occur within the heart during the cardiac cycle. A detailed description of the various abnormalities that occur in different diseases of the heart is beyond the scope of this chapter, but a few of the basic principles of recording and reading an ECG will be discussed.

Electrical basis of the ECG

Myocardial cells (**myocytes**) are capable of electrical excitation. At rest the inside of a myocardial cell (myocyte) is negatively charged with respect to the outside (Fig. 2.1). This is called the **resting potential** and in most cardiac cells measures about –90 mV.

Changes in the structure of the cell membrane lead to a sudden influx of positive charge (mainly sodium and calcium) into the cell. Within the space of a few milliseconds the electrical charge on the inside of the cell membrane changes from negative to positive and the cell is said to be **depolarized** (Fig. 2.2). The sudden change in electrical energy across the cell membrane is referred to as the **action potential** which in turn triggers myocardial contraction. Thus, mechanical activity occurs

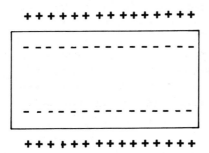

Fig. 2.1 Myocyte in the resting state. Inside of the cell is negatively charged in relation to the outside.

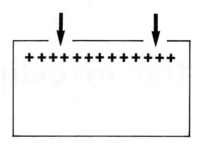

Fig. 2.2 Depolarization of the cell. Positive ions suddenly move across the membrane from outside to inside causing the action potential.

slightly after the electrical changes detected by the ECG, but only by a fraction of a second.

The heart consists of thousands of myocytes intermeshed together. They are electrically connected and so activation of one cell leads to excitation of the next and so on. Activity usually originates in the right atrium at the sino-atrial node and from here spreads out towards the apex of the heart as a **wave of depolarization** (Fig. 2.3).

This wave of depolarization spreading from one part of the heart to another means that electrical changes within the heart have both size and direction. Hence the tracing of an electrode placed in front of the advancing wave of depolarization will have a different appearance to one placed behind or at right angles. Conventionally, an impulse that moves towards an electrode registers a positive deflection. An impulse moving away from an electrode records a negative deflection, while one placed perpendicular to the direction of the impulse registers a trace that is equally positive and negative (Fig. 2.4).

Following activation of the myocyte, positive charge moves out of the cell to restore the resting potential. This is called **repolarization** and is also detected by the electrodes.

ECG leads and recording an ECG

The electrical events of depolarization and repolarization as described above may be detected on the surface of the body as the ECG. In order to record an ECG, electrodes are placed in a variety of positions and connected to an ECG machine. This converts the voltage changes associated with depolarization and repolarization into movements of a pen on a strip chart recorder. Each electrode 'views' the electrical activity of the heart from a different direction. The heart is examined in two main planes, **frontal** (coronal) and **horizontal** (transverse).

Frontal plane

The heart is examined in the frontal plane by means of electrodes placed on each limb. The electrode on the right foot is an 'earth' electrode. Each of the other electrodes generates a different 'view' of the heart called a

Direction of impulse propagation

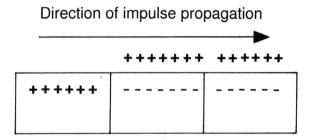

Fig. 2.3 Activation of adjacent myocytes. The action potential in the cell on the left will cause activation in the cell in the middle and, in turn, activation of the one on the right.

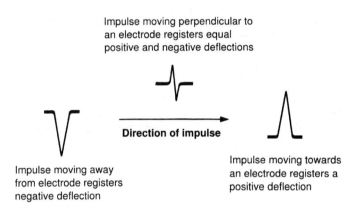

Fig. 2.4 Deflections caused by impulse propagation.

lead. The orientation of each lead in relation to the heart is given in degrees with, by convention, 0° being at 3 o'clock, +90° at six o'clock and −90° at 12 o'clock as shown in Fig. 2.5. Hence lead aVL refers to a view of the electrical activity of the heart from −30°; aVF from +90° and aVR from −150°. Leads aVL, aVR and aVF are called **unipolar leads** as they compare the electrical activity of a certain electrode to zero. (The 'a' stands for **'augmented'**. The limb leads are quite some distance from the heart so the electrical changes that they pick up are correspondingly small. The machine compensates for this by 'augmenting' the voltages detected).

Because each 'view' of the heart has both size and direction it is possible to generate different views by adding and subtracting different combinations of electrodes. **Standard leads I, II and III** are called **bipolar** leads as they compare the electrical signals from two electrodes (rather than from a single electrode against zero as with unipolar leads). They

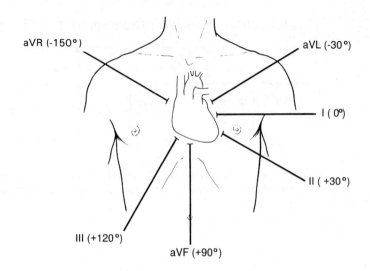

Fig. 2.5 Orientation of ECG leads to the heart in the frontal plane. It can be seen that leads II, III and aVF examine mainly the inferior wall of the heart and leads I and aVL the high lateral wall.

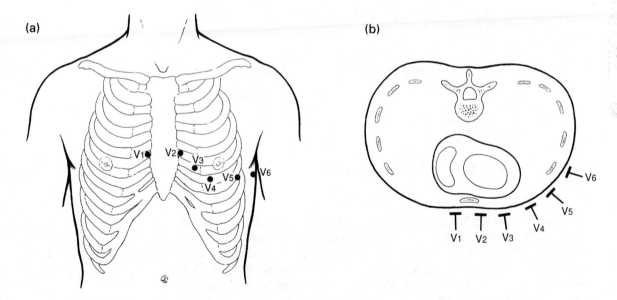

Fig. 2.6 Orientation of chest leads to the heart. (a) On the anterior chest wall. (b) In transverse section.

are effectively different 'views' of the heart created by the machine and their orientation to the heart is shown in Fig. 2.5. It can be seen that lead I refers to a view of the electrical activity of the heart from 0° (3 o'clock), lead II from +30° and lead III from +120°. It is not important to know how each lead is calculated, but if the electrodes are connected incorrectly the machine will add/subtract the wrong leads and the ECG will be uninterpretable.

Horizontal plane

The heart is examined in the horizontal (transverse) plane using six electrodes placed at intervals around the anterior chest wall. They are called the **chest leads** and are numbered V_{1-6}. Their positioning in relation to the heart is shown in Fig. 2.6. Although the RV lies below V_{1-2} its thin wall means it contributes little to the electrical activity of the heart. Thus these leads are useful mainly for examining the **interventricular septum**. V_{3-4} are useful for the anterior LV wall and V_{5-6} examine mainly the lateral wall of the LV.

Heart rate and the ECG

Paper in the ECG machine moves at a standard rate of 25 mm/s. By measuring the number of squares between complexes it is possible to calculate the heart rate. Each large square on the ECG paper represents 0.2 s. A large square consists of five small squares, so each of these represents 0.04 s. There are several methods for calculating heart rate and each person usually has their own preferred one. Two examples are given below.

One QRS complex per large square is equivalent to a heart rate of 300/min. (each large square is 0.2 s, so there are 5/s and 300/min.). One QRS every two squares therefore represents a rate of 150/min; one every three squares a rate of 100/min and so on. In short, the heart rate is 300 divided by the number of large squares between each QRS (Fig. 2.7). This method assumes that the heart rate is regular and the distance between successive QRS complexes is constant.

(a)

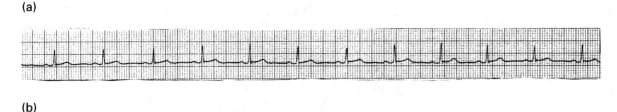

(b)

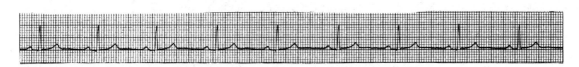

Fig. 2.7 Rhythm strips. (a) There is a QRS complex every four large squares, so the rate is 300/4 = 75. (b) There is a QRS complex every five large squares, so the rate is 300/5 = 60.

An alternative, quick, method is to use the 'rhythm strip' that is printed at the bottom of most standard ECG recordings. This is a longer recording of a particular lead and is included in the printout to help with the diagnosis of rhythm disorders. A rhythm strip is a 10s recording. Counting the number of QRS complexes in a 10s rhythm strip and multiplying by 6 will give the heart rate in beats/min.

Voltage deflections and calibration

The size of a deflection on the ECG is only useful if it can be compared to the deflection caused by a known voltage change. An electrical signal of 1 mV should cause a deflection of 1 cm (two large squares) on the ECG paper. Using this calibration it is possible to translate the size of a deflection into a voltage and infer information about the magnitude of the underlying electrical activity of the heart.

Electrical 'wiring' of the heart

In order to understand the various deflections seen on the ECG it is first necessary to recap the electrical 'wiring' system of the heart. All myocardial cells are able to generate their own action potentials spontaneously. However, a group of cells located high up in the right atrium, the **sino-atrial (SA) node**, have the fastest rate of self-depolaization and therefore dictate the heart rate under most circumstances.

From the sinus node depolarization spreads throughout both atria. The atria and ventricles are separated by a fibrous ring which is

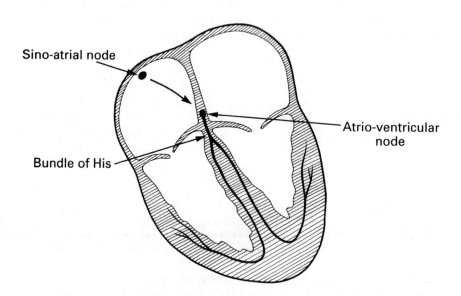

Fig. 2.8 The 'electrical wiring' of the heart.

electrically inactive. Communication is therefore through a narrow strand of specialized heart tissue called the **atrio-ventricular (AV) node** which lies low down in the atrial septum and traverses the fibrous ring (Fig. 2.8). At the top of the ventricular septum this cord of conducting tissue (now called the Bundle of His) divides into two. The daughter strands are called the **right and left bundles**. The left bundle divides again into two **fascicles**, termed **anterior** and **posterior**. All of these strands of conducting tissue run in the septum. It is important to realize that these cords of electrical tissue are extremely small. Damage to one or more of them significantly alters the connections between the atria and the ventricles and causes characteristic changes in the tracings recorded by the ECG. The right bundle and the two fascicles then undergo multiple divisions into a diffuse network of activating fibres. These are called **His Purkinje fibres** and they provide a quick and efficient mechanism for the uniform activation of ventricular muscle.

Deflections recorded by the ECG

The heart consists of many interlaced cells, but for the purposes of understanding the ECG it is helpful to consider it as two separate units: atria and ventricles. The fibrous ring that separates the atria from the ventricles means that electrical events in these two areas are distinct. Figure 2.9 shows the different deflections of the ECG.

P wave

From the SA node, depolarization spreads rapidly throughout both atria. The mass of muscle in the atria is relatively small and so the deflection produced by its depolarization is also relatively small. It is called the P wave and usually measures <2.5 mV in amplitude and lasts not longer than 0.08 s (two small squares). Normal P wave morphology is shown in Fig. 2.9 and is produced when excitation spreads from the SA node through normal-sized atria with normal conduction properties. Hence abnormal P waves may be produced when the size of the atrium is abnormal or if depolarization does not originate in the sinus node.

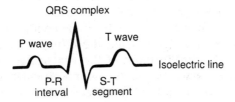

Fig. 2.9 The normal ECG complex.

P–R interval

Following atrial depolarization there follows a period when propagation of the electrical impulse is slightly delayed. This period is called the P–R interval and represents the time taken for the impulse to move down through the AV node (which conducts relatively slowly) and into the specialized ventricular conduction system. In normal people the P–R interval lasts 0.12–0.2 s (three to five small squares). Under certain conditions the AV node conducts less efficiently and the P–R interval may be longer than 0.2 s. Sometimes an impulse never 'gets through' and a P wave occurs on its own. These and other aspects of conduction disease are discussed in Chapter 6.

QRS complex

This refers to the deflections created when depolarization spreads through the ventricles. Impulses are conducted to the ventricles by the His Purkinje system so ventricular depolarization is efficient and is

---

Terminology of the QRS complex

Because of the different views that each lead has of electrical activity in the heart each QRS complex looks different in each lead. It is important therefore to be able to identify each component of the QRS complex.

1. If the initial deflection in the QRS complex is negative it is called a **q wave**. Normal q waves last no longer than 0.04 s (one small square) and should be no deeper than 25% of the height of the following positive deflection. Negative deflections that are wider and/or deeper than this are said to be **pathological** and are termed **Q waves**. They are usually the result of myocardial infarction and are discussed in the chapter on ischaemic heart disease. The exception to this is lead aVR where Q waves are quite normal.
2. The positive component of the QRS complex is called the **R wave**. It may or may not be preceded by a negative deflection.
3. The **S wave** refers to a negative deflection after an R wave.

---

complete within 0.12 s (three small squares). If the QRS complex is wider than this it usually suggests either that there is damage to the His Purkinje system causing delayed ventricular activation, or that ventricular depolarization has not been via the conduction system at all.

For the purposes of understanding the different deflections of the QRS complex it is helpful to think of the ventricular muscle as being composed of three separate masses: the interventricular septum, the free wall of the right ventricle and the free wall of the left ventricle. Figure 2.10 shows a cross-section through the heart with the three muscle masses shaded in.

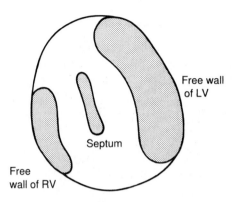

Fig. 2.10 Cross-section through the heart showing the free wall of the right ventricle, interventricular septum and free wall of the left ventricle.

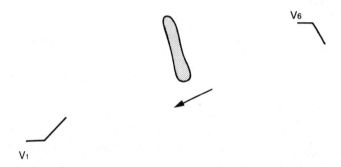

Fig. 2.11 Septal depolarization is from left to right causing a small positive deflection in V₁ and a small negative deflection in V₆.

As impulses travel through the conduction pathways it is the **septum** that depolarizes first. The left bundle is activated slightly earlier than the right bundle and so the septum itself is activated from left to right, as shown in Fig. 2.11. As a result of septal depolarization, leads that overlie the right ventricle (such as V_1) register an initial positive deflection. Leads that examine the left ventricle (such as V_6) register a negative deflection. The mass of muscle in the septum is small and so both of these deflections are correspondingly small.

Following septal depolarization impulses spread throughout both ventricles simultaneously. There is more muscle in the left ventricle than the right ventricle, so the overall direction of depolarization is to the left. Hence even those leads that overlie the right ventricle will detect mainly the effect of left ventricular depolarization and register a negative deflection (Fig. 2.12). Between V_1 and V_6 there is a gradual transition from negative deflections to positive ones, as shown in Fig. 2.13.

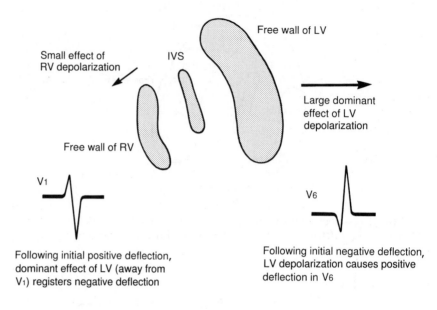

Small effect of RV depolarization

IVS

Free wall of LV

Large dominant effect of LV depolarization

Free wall of RV

V₁

V₆

Following initial positive deflection, dominant effect of LV (away from V₁) registers negative deflection

Following initial negative deflection, LV depolarization causes positive deflection in V₆

Fig. 2.12 Depolarization of the free wall of the left ventricle causes characteristic deflections in the chest leads.

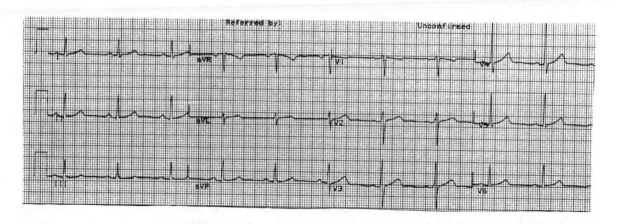

Fig. 2.13 Normal 12-lead ECG.

T wave

The T wave is the electrical recording that accompanies ventricular repolarization. The T wave should be positive if the preceding QRS is positive and negative if the QRS is negative. A wide variety of structural, mechanical, electrical and metabolic conditions may cause changes in the morphology of T waves and so care should be exercised before ascribing any T wave abnormality to a particular cardiac pathology.

S–T segment

This refers to the portion of the ECG that lies between the end of the QRS complex and the onset of the T wave. It should be flat and **isoelectric** (on the baseline). The S–T segment may deviate from the isoelectric line in normal individuals (particularly black Africans), but more commonly this is associated with underlying cardiac disease.

Cardiac axis

Each cell, when activated, generates its own little impulse that has a certain size and direction. Myocytes are arranged together in a criss-cross fashion, so impulses moving in opposite directions will, in effect, cancel each other out. However, because the general direction of movement of the wave of depolarization is from the SA node (top right of the heart) to the apex (bottom left) there is an overall direction of propagation of the electrical impulse which is the net result of adding together the thousands of mini-impulses produced by each myocyte. This is called the **cardiac axis**. It is calculated using the leads that examine the heart in the frontal plane so it is also known as the **mean frontal axis**. It is conventional to quote the direction of the cardiac axis in degrees, with 0° being at 3 o'clock. Numbers progress clockwise, so that +90° is at 6 o'clock and –90° at 12 o'clock.

The cardiac axis can be calculated from the relative size of the positive and negative deflections in the six frontal leads of the ECG. A convenient way is to find the lead with the smallest, most equiphasic complexes. The cardiac axis will be approximately at right angles to this, as shown in Fig. 2.14.

In the example shown in Fig. 2.15, the equiphasic complex in aVF (+90°) suggests that the axis must either be 0° or 180°. Lead I is all positive and lead III mainly negative so the axis must be 0°.

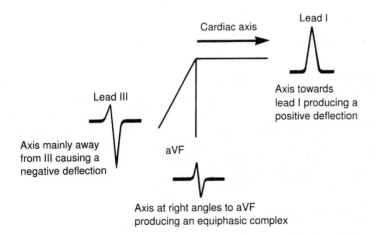

Fig. 2.14 Calculating the cardiac axis.

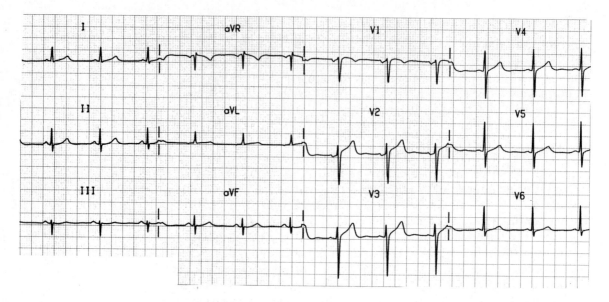

Fig. 2.15 In this ECG the complexes are equiphasic in aVF, so the axis is at right angles to this lead. Lead I is all positive so the axis must be 0°.

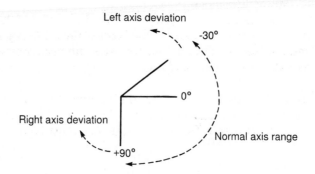

Fig. 2.16 Axis deviation.

A normal axis lies between −30° and +90° (Fig. 2.16). An axis 'more anti-clockwise' than −30° is referred to as **left axis deviation** and one 'more clockwise' than +90° is called **right axis deviation**. A full description of the causes of axis deviation will not be given here. The important principle to understand is that interruption of the normal conduction pathways and alterations in the relative proportions of left and right ventricular muscle may both cause axis shift.

Abnormal QRS complexes

QRS morphology may be abnormal in size or shape. Widening of the QRS complex (>0.12 s) suggests either that conduction through the His

Purkinje system has been disrupted (**bundle branch block**) or that depolarization has originated in the ventricular muscle itself rather than the conduction system. Both are discussed in Chapter 6.

Abnormally large deflections may occur when the amount of muscle undergoing depolarization is increased. The commonest cardiac chamber to increase in size is the left ventricle (LV) and this is called **left ventricular hypertrophy**. From Fig. 2.6 it can be seen that the leads that examine the LV are mainly V_5 and V_6. In addition it will be remembered that the negative deflection in leads V_1 and V_2 is due to the greater muscle mass of the LV overriding the effect of the smaller right ventricle (RV). In LV hypertrophy this dominant effect is even more pronounced and leads V_1 and V_2 register a very deep negative deflection (S wave). V_5 and V_6 both register very large positive deflections (R waves). If the height of the R wave in V_6 + the depth of the S wave in V_1 is greater than or equals 35 mm then this suggests LV hypertrophy. However, the ECG is a relatively insensitive tool for making this diagnosis, as the voltages may be higher in thin people and lower in fat people. The echocardiogram is able to measure the thickness of the LV wall and is a more sensitive investigation for detecting LV hypertrophy.

24-Hour ambulatory monitoring (Holter monitoring)

This is most frequently used in the investigation of patients with suspected arrhythmias. It involves the continuous monitoring of two or more ECG leads by a small recorder the size of a personal stereo attached to the patient. Patients keep a diary of their symptoms (such as palpitation, syncope or pre-syncope) so that the timing of these may be related to the timing of any arrhythmias detected by the machine.

Exercise testing

Many patients with cardiological problems develop symptoms only on exertion and the resting ECG is often completely normal. Exercise testing is an investigation that aims to reproduce those symptoms under controlled, supervised conditions and document any ECG abnormalities that occur. It is most often used in the diagnosis of coronary artery disease. The patient exercises on a sloping treadmill or bicycle according to a graded protocol and is instructed to report any symptoms. The ECG and blood pressure are recorded throughout. A positive test is said to occur if there is 1 mm or more of horizontal or downsloping S–T segment depression in one or more leads of the ECG. If there are ECG changes suggestive of ischaemia after only a little exercise it suggests that the narrowings in the coronary arteries are severe. Most such patients should be investigated further with coronary angiography in order to define the coronary anatomy and plan further management.

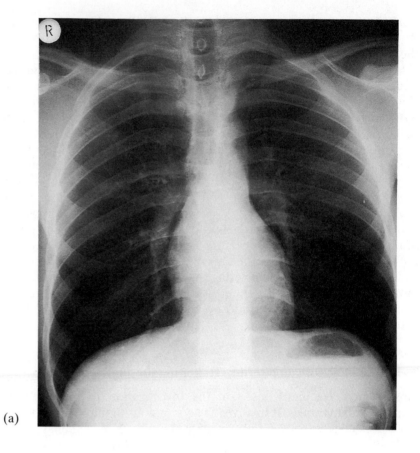

(a)

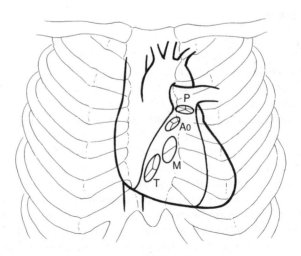

(b)

Fig. 2.17 (a) Normal chest X-ray with (b) a diagram of the surface projections.

CHEST X-RAY

A diagram of the surface projection of the heart and great vessels is shown together with a normal chest X-ray (Fig. 2.17). From these it can be seen that:

1. The right heart border is created mainly by the right atrium and superior vena cava.
2. The left heart border is made up of the left ventricle and left atrium.
3. The apex of the heart points slightly downwards and is medial to the midclavicular line.
4. The right ventricle sits on the diaphragm.

Cardiac silhouette

The heart is situated anteriorly in the chest so an X-ray taken with the chest against the film (PA) minimizes the degree of magnification (and therefore distortion) of the cardiac structures.

Size

The ratio of transverse diameter of the heart : transverse diameter of the thorax is called the cardiothoracic ratio (**CTR**). In normal people the CTR is 0.5 or less. A CTR of greater than 0.5 suggests that the heart is enlarged (called cardiomegaly) and is usually the result of dilatation of one or both ventricles or a pericardial effusion. Hypertrophy alone rarely increases the size of the cardiac silhouette.

Shape

Enlargement of particular cardiac chambers often causes characteristic alterations in the shape of the cardiac shadow.

Left atrial enlargement (Fig. 2.18)
This is commonly the result of mitral valve disease and may cause three abnormalities which can be understood with an appreciation of some simple anatomy. First, the left atrium (LA) forms the upper part of the left heart border and this is usually concave upwards. If the LA is enlarged this concavity becomes flattened and may even become convex upwards. Second, the LA lies mainly posteriorly and so as the atrium enlarges it does so behind the ventricles. This creates an extra shadow on the X-ray next to the right heart border, which appears to have a double outline. Third, the LA sits under the bifurcation of the trachea (the carina). Enlargement of the LA pushes the two main bronchi apart, with the left main bronchus becoming more horizontal and the carina becomes more splayed.

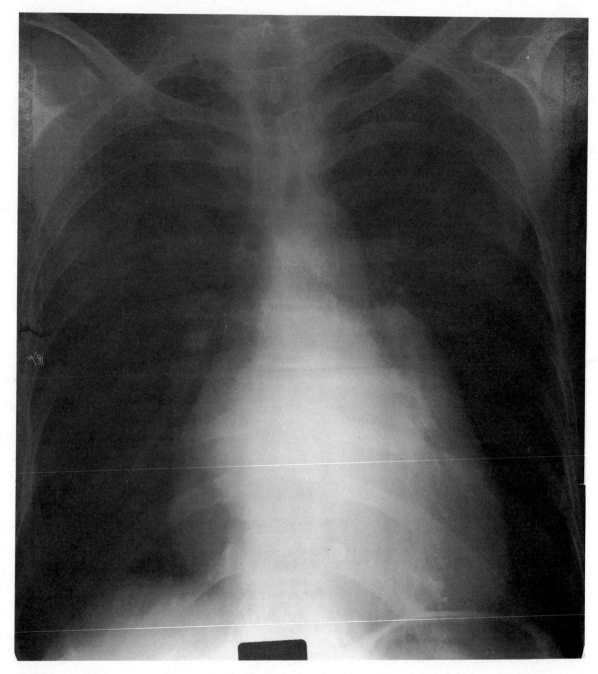

Fig. 2.18 Left atrial enlargement. Note the 'double shadow' at the right heart border and the bulging of the left heart border below the pulmonary artery.

Right ventricular enlargement (Fig. 2.19)
The RV sits mainly on the surface of the diaphragm. When it enlarges it pushes the apex of the heart upwards and to the left. The right heart border may become more prominent but this is often hard to appreciate on the CXR.

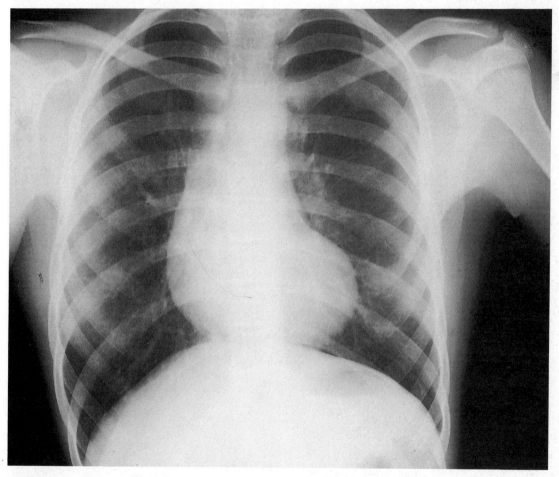

Fig. 2.19   Right ventricular enlargement. The apex is lifted 'up and to the left'.

Left ventricular enlargement (Fig. 2.20)
The LV forms most of the left heart border. When it enlarges it usually pushes the apex laterally and inferiorly and the CTR is increased.

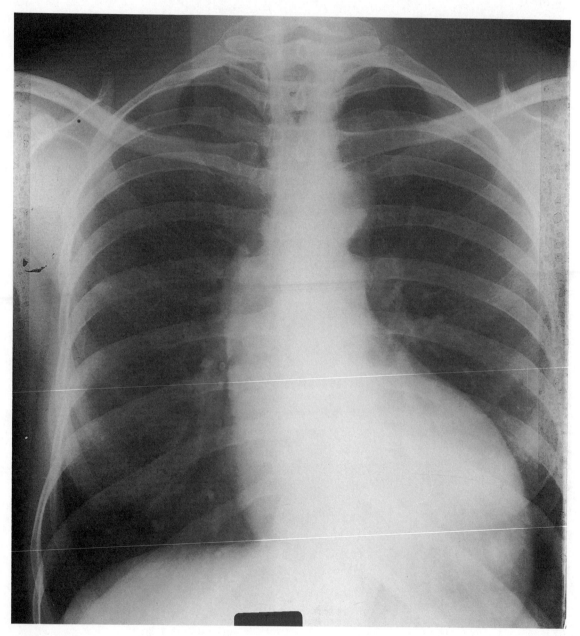

Fig. 2.20   Left ventricular enlargement. The apex is pushed laterally and inferiorly.

Lateral chest X-ray

When cardiomegaly is noted it may be difficult to decide which ventricle is primarily responsible. The lateral chest X-ray is extremely helpful under these circumstances. The RV lies more anteriorly than the LV so enlargement of this chamber will shrink the **retrosternal** space on the lateral view. By contrast LV enlargement reduces the size of the **retrocardiac** space (Fig. 2.21).

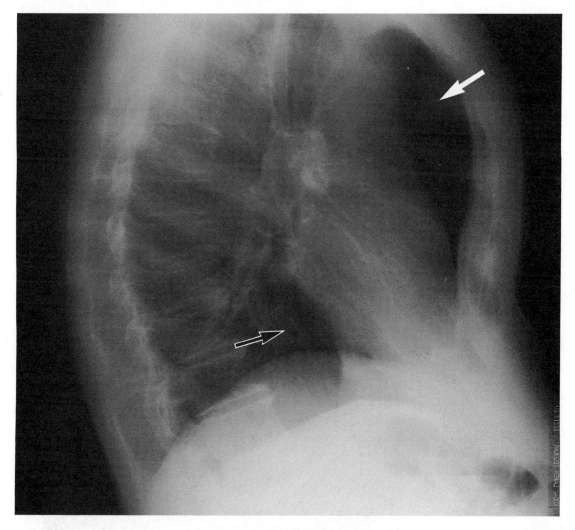

Fig. 2.21   Normal lateral chest X-ray with retrosternal (solid) and retrocardiac (hollow) spaces arrowed.

ECHOCARDIOGRAPHY

This technique uses ultrasound to gain information about the structure and function of the heart. Sound waves pass through different soft tissues (such as muscle and blood) at approximately the same rate, but at points where the tissue density changes (such as the interface between a cardiac chamber and blood) some of the sound waves are reflected. A piezo-electric crystal within the ultrasound probe is able to emit and detect sound waves and use this information to construct an image of the heart. The images are presented in one of two ways. In **M** (for 'Motion') **Mode** the ultrasound beam is fixed along a certain line. With movement of the heart in systole and diastole the beam finds the tissue interfaces at different positions and from this the machine is able to derive information about changes in cardiac dimensions with time. In **2-D echo** an arc of sound waves (rather than a linear beam) is directed from the probe which produces a cross-sectional image of the heart (Fig. 2.22).

Doppler echocardiography

The Doppler effect refers to the change in the pitch of a note that occurs when the sound source moves relative to the listener. An everyday example of this occurs when an ambulance drives past. The note from the siren gets higher as the ambulance approaches and becomes deeper as it recedes into the distance. In the context of echocardiography the Doppler effect refers to the change in the pattern of sound waves detected with different velocities of blood flow. If a valve is narrowed

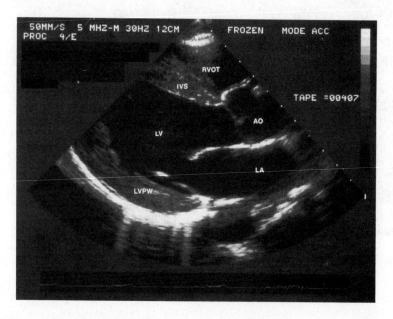

Fig. 2.22 Parasternal view of the heart on echocardiography.

(stenosed) then flow across the valve must be faster if the same volume of blood is to be ejected in the same period of time. The Doppler probe is able to detect these abnormal flow patterns associated with **stenosed valves** and also identify abnormal **regurgitant jets**.

Transoesophageal echocardiography

Because bone and lung tissue are relatively poor conductors of ultrasound it is not always possible to obtain high quality images from studies with the probe placed on the chest wall. **Transoesophageal echocardiography** involves the use of an ultrasound probe mounted on an endoscope. This means that the heart is much closer to the ultrasound source and the sound waves have less tissue and no bone or lung to pass through. The images obtained, particularly of posterior heart structures such as the left atrium and the aorta, are of excellent quality.

Echocardiography is the most useful non-invasive technique for obtaining information about chamber dimensions, valve motion, left ventricular function and for identifying pericardial effusions.

NUCLEAR CARDIOLOGY

In recent years techniques that involve the use of radiolabelled isotopes have become increasingly used. They provide information about the function of the heart and the two most commonly used tests are technetium and thallium scanning.

^{99}Technetium-labelled nuclear angiography

In this technique the blood is made temporarily radioactive with the isotope ^{99}technetium. A gamma camera is then placed over the chest to detect the level of radioactivity in the blood as it circulates through the heart. A computer then processes the data to construct an image of the heart. Two different studies can be made, both of which provide similar information. In the **first pass method** the level of radioactivity is measured during the first circulation through the heart of an intravenous bolus of isotope. In the **equilibrium method** the red blood cells are labelled with ^{99}technetium and counting begins only after the bolus of isotope has had time to become evenly distributed throughout the whole circulation.

An ECG is recorded as the computer acquires data. By measuring the different amounts of radioactivity at different points in the cardiac cycle the computer is able to calculate how much of the blood present in the LV at the end of diastole (called the end-diastolic volume) is ejected during systole. This is called the **ejection fraction** and is an important determinant of prognosis in cardiac disease. Sometimes a portion of myocardium moves normally at rest but less well when the heart is stressed by exercise and this can be visualized by nuclear angiography. This is called a **regional wall abnormality** and is usually due to coronary artery disease. A narrowed coronary artery is unable to increase its delivery of blood during exercise and the portion of muscle supplied by that artery becomes ischaemic. As a result it moves less well than at rest and this can be detected on the nuclear angiogram.

^{201}Thallium scintigraphy

This technique relies on the fact that the radioisotope ^{201}Thallium (a potassium analogue) is taken up by myocardial cells. If the blood supply to the heart is uniform then following an intravenous bolus of this isotope a gamma camera placed over the chest will detect a homo-geneous distribution of the isotope throughout the heart. Intravenous dipyridamole or adenosene are coronary vasodilators that dilate normal arteries more than diseased vessels. Hence following their injection, thallium will be taken up preferentially by myocardium served by normal arteries and less well in areas supplied by diseased arteries. Four hours later the scan is repeated, following 'redistribution' of thallium throughout the heart. If the distribution of isotope becomes homogeneous it suggests that the original perfusion defect was a reversible one. This is usually due to coronary artery disease. If the perfusion defect is still seen it suggests that the area of myocardium is permanently damaged, usually due to infarction.

CARDIAC CATHETERIZATION AND CORONARY ANGIOGRAPHY

Catheterization is the term given to the insertion of tubes into cavities of the body for the purposes of introducing and withdrawing fluids or measuring pressures. In the context of cardiac disease it is an invaluable method of obtaining information about the anatomy and function of the chambers and vessels of the heart. **Coronary angiography** is the study of the anatomy of the coronary vessels. Although the details of the procedure vary according to whether the right or left heart or coronary arteries are being studied, the principles of cardiac catheterization are similar and involve the introduction, percutaneously, of a fine tube into either an artery (for the study of the left heart and coronary arteries) or a vein (for the right heart and pulmonary arteries). The catheter is then fed round to the chamber or vessel to be studied.

The study of the anatomy of the coronary vessels involves the introduction of a catheter into the left side of the heart. This may be done by exposing the brachial artery under local anaesthetic or, more commonly, by cannulating the femoral artery using the **Seldinger technique**. Here a needle is inserted into the femoral artery, followed by a guide wire threaded through its lumen. The needle is removed and a sheath with a one way valve is fed over the wire into the artery.

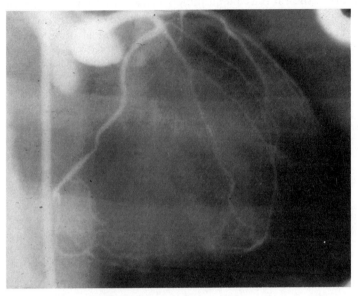

Fig. 2.23   Normal left coronary arteriogram.

Pre-shaped catheters may then be fed into the femoral artery, up the aorta and into the left and right coronary arteries. Injection of radio-opaque contrast outlines the coronary artery anatomy (Fig. 2.23). Each major coronary vessel is studied in turn and abnormalities of anatomy are usually described in terms of the degree of narrowing (stenosis), such as 70% stenosis of the left anterior descending artery. The number of narrowings seen at angiography is variable. Disease may be confined to one artery only or involve all three main vessels (triple vessel disease). Assessment of left ventricular function is made by placing a catheter in the LV. Contrast is injected rapidly through multiple side holes in the catheter which outlines the movement of the ventricular wall as it contracts.

Electrophysiological studies

This involves the use of electrodes placed inside the heart to study the pattern and timing of electrical activity. Recordings are usually made from the region of the sinus node, bundle of His, right ventricle and sometimes the coronary sinus (which measures left atrial and ventricular activity). In addition to generating a detailed map of the electrical activity of the heart in sinus rhythm it is often possible to induce arrhythmias by delivering extra stimuli to the right atrium or right ventricle. This may help in the diagnosis of symptoms such as syncope or, if the arrhythmia induced correlates with a previously documented arrhythmia, the patient may be retested after administration of various anti-arrhythmic drugs. If the drug(s) prevents the induction of tachycardia then it may be suitable for use as a long-term prophylactic agent. Accessory electrical pathways between the atria and ventricles which cause tachycardias may be mapped and destroyed ('ablated').

Heart failure | 3

Cardiac failure is a condition that is diagnosed with accuracy and consistency by most doctors, but is difficult to define. It may be thought of as 'a syndrome in which, despite normal or raised venous pressures, the heart is unable to maintain an adequate circulation and meet the requirements of metabolizing tissues'. Hypovolaemic states such as acute haemorrhage are therefore excluded as causes of heart failure, because in these cases cardiac output is low chiefly as a result of poor venous return. In the past confusion has arisen because conditions of so-called 'high output' cardiac failure have been included in the definition. In these conditions the heart is unable to maintain an adequate circulation because the metabolic demands of the tissues are so high. Cardiac function is otherwise normal. This chapter will focus on causes of cardiac failure in which there is a demonstrable abnormality of the heart.

PHYSIOLOGICAL ASPECTS

Cardiac output is the product of stroke volume (the amount of blood ejected with each contraction) and heart rate. Stroke volume, in turn, is governed by the **force** of myocardial contraction and by the pre- and afterload demands placed on the heart. **Afterload** refers to the resistance against which the ventricle must contract. **Hypertension** (in which there is increased resistance to blood flow) and **aortic stenosis** (in which the outlet of the left ventricle is obstructed) are common causes of increased afterload which may eventually result in impaired myocardial performance. **Preload** refers to the amount of force (or stretch) that myocardial fibres undergo during diastolic relaxation. In the context of understanding heart failure it is sometimes useful to think of preload as referring to the pressure within the ventricles at the end of diastolic filling. This is chiefly a function of the venous return to the heart, which in turn is dependent on the pressure in the venous system.

The rapidly changing demands placed on the heart with such factors as exercise, temperature and hormonal environment requires a virtually instantaneous method of adjusting cardiac output. This is the essence of the **Starling law of the heart**, which states that at fixed levels of myocardial contractility, stroke volume is proportional to changes in

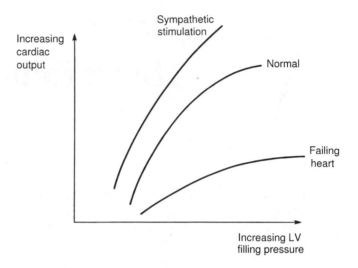

Fig. 3.1 Starling curves. Increases in preload (filling pressure) give rise to significant increases in cardiac output in normal and sympathetically stimulated hearts. With a failing heart large increases in preload cause comparatively little increase in cardiac output.

preload (i.e. changes in the stretch of myocardial fibres). In clinical terms, therefore, Starling's law may be taken to mean that an increase in venous return (and therefore pressure) will cause an increase in cardiac output, as shown in Fig. 3.1.

The altered haemodynamic forces that result from a fall in cardiac output invoke a series of compensatory changes, some of which are appropriate and some of which are more suited to hypovolaemic states such as blood loss. They include a rise in venous pressures, fluid retention, peripheral vasoconstriction and changes in heart shape.

Venous pressures

With impaired myocardial function the amount of blood ejected with each contraction falls and the volume of blood remaining in the ventricle at the end of systole increases. During diastole more blood arrives for the next contraction. Together, this means that pressure in the ventricle at the end of diastole (called the **end diastolic pressure, EDP**) is increased. Part of the body's response to a fall in cardiac output is constriction of the large veins in an attempt to divert blood centrally, increase venous return and improve cardiac output along the Starling curve. However, with a failing myocardium, the ventricular function curve is set lower than normal (Fig. 3.1), so that increases in preload give rise to increases in stroke volume that are less than those predicted from the normal Starling curve. In advanced heart failure the ventricular function curve is virtually flat so that, despite large venous filling pressures and tachycardia, cardiac output is low. It is this combination of a high EDP and raised venous pressures that are partly responsible for some of the symptoms of cardiac failure.

Salt and water retention

This arises chiefly out of the response of the renal cortex to hypoperfusion. The impaired pumping action of the heart leads to a fall in glomerular filtration rate. The reduced flow of sodium and chloride in the distal tubule activates the **renin–angiotensin–aldosterone system**

Renin–angiotensin–aldosterone system

This system provides a homeostatic mechanism by which body salt, plasma volume and blood pressure are regulated. **Renin (a proteolytic enzyme)** is released by the juxta-glomerular cells of the renal cortex in response either to decreased pressures in the efferent arteriole or to falling concentrations of sodium chloride in the distal nephron. Renin acts on a globular protein present in plasma, forming the decapeptide **angiotensin I (AT I)**. AT I has no physiological action and is converted to **AT II** by **angiotensin converting enzyme (ACE)**, found mainly in lung. AT II has two important physiological actions. First, it is a powerful **vasoconstrictor** of arterioles and veins. Second, it stimulates the adrenal cortex to secrete the hormone **aldosterone**, which in turn acts on receptors in the distal tubule to promote salt and water retention. As a response to hypovolaemia, activation of the renin–angiotensin system is entirely appropriate, but in the context of heart failure with fluid overload it exacerbates the high venous pressures that ultimately cause symptoms.

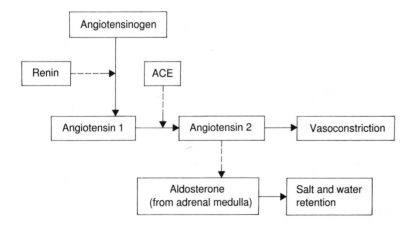

Fig. 3.2 The renin–angiotensin system in heart failure causing vasoconstriction and salt and water retention.

in an effort to retain salt and water (Fig. 3.2). Such a response would be appropriate to acute blood loss (in order to maintain intravascular volume) but, set in the context of heart failure with high venous pressures, leads to fluid overload.

Vasoconstriction

This is probably due to a baroreceptor reflex designed to maintain blood pressure and safeguard cerebral and renal perfusion in the face of falling cardiac output. Arteriolar vasoconstriction causes increased peripheral resistance to blood flow. This increases the afterload against which the dysfunctioning left ventricle must contract, worsening cardiac performance still further. Vasoconstriction is also mediated by increased activity of the renin–angiotensin system.

Changes in heart shape

As the heart fails the ventricles are less able to empty themselves and the heart begins to **dilate**. If the heart were operating on the normal Starling curve an increase in end-diastolic pressure (preload) would improve cardiac output. However, with the flat curve that exists in heart failure high pressures lead to pulmonary and systemic congestion.

If the afterload demands on the heart are very high the ventricle responds by increasing its muscle mass. This is called **hypertrophy** and is most important in hypertension and aortic stenosis, where there is increased resistance to ventricular emptying. Hypertrophy also occurs in response to ventricular dilatation but is less marked.

Heart failure: compensatory changes

Increased venous pressure
Salt and water retention
Vasoconstriction
Changes in heart shape (hypertrophy/dilatation)

CLINICAL PATTERNS OF HEART FAILURE

The clinical features of heart failure are due to a combination of salt and water retention leading to fluid overload; high venous pressures due to the falling output of the failing ventricle; and generalized underperfusion of organs. It is useful in heart failure to divide the clinical features into two groups, although it should be remembered that they frequently occur together.

Left ventricular failure

Acute left ventricular failure (LVF)

Sudden deteriorations in left ventricular function are usually the result of myocardial infarction. There is less muscle available for contraction so cardiac output falls. Reflex activation of the sympathetic autonomic nervous system leads to tachycardia and peripheral vasoconstriction in an attempt to maintain blood pressure and protect vital organs from underperfusion. Incomplete emptying of the left ventricle means that pressures within this chamber at the end of diastole (**left ventricular end-diastolic pressures**) are high. These high pressures feed back to the pulmonary vasculature and fluid seeps into the alveoli. This gives rise to the main symptom of acute LVF which is **severe breathlessness**, sometimes associated with the production of pink frothy sputum.

Chronic left ventricular failure

Here, the decline in myocardial performance takes place over months or years. As discussed earlier this fall-off in cardiac output results in high venous pressures, vasoconstriction and fluid retention. The insidious rise in venous pressures on the left side of the heart alters the balance of the hydrostatic and oncotic pressures in the post capillary venule. Fluid

---

Effort dyspnoea

The precise physiological explanation for breathlessness on exercise is much disputed. Previously it was thought that a rise in right ventricular output with exercise caused accumulation of fluid in the lungs as the left ventricle was unable to increase its output. However, there are several lines of evidence to dispute this. First, if poor ventricular function is the underlying cause of effort dyspnoea, then severity of exercise limitation should correlate with the extent of ventricular dysfunction but this is not the case. Second, one might expect LA filling pressure to correlate with the end of symptom limited exercise but this is not so. Third, if high left atrial pressures are to blame for the symptoms of breathlessness, one would expect correction of this abnormality by cardiac transplantation to bring about an immediate improvement in symptoms. Studies show that it takes several weeks for the full benefit of transplantation to be seen.

Many authorities believe that **metabolic changes** in skeletal muscle are important in the symptoms of dyspnoea. Blood flow to skeletal muscle is reduced in heart failure so that, with exercise, a metabolic acidosis develops. Peripheral chemoreceptors trigger a hyperventilatory response, causing a sensation of breathlessness.

Symptoms of left heart failure

Breathlessness with exercise
Orthopnoea
Paroxysmal nocturnal dyspnoea
Tiredness, fatigue

---

seeps into the pulmonary interstitium, causing breathlessness on exercise (effort dyspnoea). As fluid congestion in the lungs worsens the symptom of breathlessness may occur at rest, particularly when lying flat. This is called **orthopnoea**. Patients who experience this symptom frequently make use of extra pillows at night to help them sleep in a more upright position. Some patients experience breathlessness at night in the form of **paroxysmal nocturnal dyspnoea (PND)**. A typical episode of PND involves waking at night breathless with a sensation of being suffocated, sometimes accompanied by sweating. Often the patient will feel the need to open a window and breathe fresh air. Orthopnoea and PND are both features of an over-expanded circulation caused by salt and water retention. It is the change from the horizontal to upright position that relieves the symptom of breathlessness as pressures in the pulmonary veins become lowered.

Signs of left heart failure are due to a combination of pulmonary congestion and oedema (fine crepitations in the lung bases) and cardiac 'distress' at the abnormal haemodynamic loads (added heart sounds). With more severe left ventricular failure the signs become more marked. The 'gallop rhythm' is a classic sign of severe heart failure and is caused by the summated 3rd and 4th heart sounds at fast heart rates (Chapter 1). There may also be signs of reflex activation of the sympathetic autonomic nervous system (tachycardia with sweaty, clammy skin and

---

Heart failure in lung disease

The arrangement of the systemic and pulmonary circulations in series means that changes in the functioning of one system may cause haemodynamic upset in the other. Primary lung pathology, either acute or chronic, affects the functioning of the right ventricle and may eventually cause right heart failure. The commonest cause of increased pulmonary resistance is chronic obstructive airways disease (COAD). The permanent state of hypoxia, together with carbon dioxide retention and acidosis causes chronic vasoconstriction of the pulmonary arterioles. Increased pulmonary vascular resistance leads to pulmonary hypertension. This increases the afterload on the right ventricle, compromising its function until eventually it fails and dilates. RV failure secondary to lung disease is called **cor pulmonale**.

Symptoms of right heart failure

Ankle swelling
Tiredness, fatigue
Breathlessness with exercise
Abdominal swelling
Right upper quadrant discomfort

---

peripheral shutdown) as blood is diverted towards the vital organs in order to safeguard their perfusion.

Right ventricular failure

Most cases of right heart failure occur as a consequence of left heart failure. Isolated right heart failure is usually due to an increased afterload on the right ventricle (RV) which may develop acutely or over several years. Sudden increases in resistance to right ventricular output occur in **pulmonary embolism**, where there is obstruction to blood flow by clot in the pulmonary circulation. Examples in which increased resistance takes place over a longer period include recurrent, smaller pulmonary emboli and the pulmonary hypertension that accompanies longstanding chronic obstructive airways disease.

Case history
A 58-year-old man presented to his GP with ankle swelling. He was a regular attender at the surgery to collect prescriptions for antibiotics and inhalers for his frequent attacks of 'winter bronchitis' which he blamed on 40 years of heavy smoking. Despite these he was able to continue working as a hotel lift operator, but in the previous few months had had increasing difficulty putting on his shoes. On examination his fingers were nicotine-stained and he was barrel chested. The venous pressure was elevated to 10 cm above the sternal angle and there were obvious systolic pulsations in its waveform. There was pitting oedema to the mid calf. Palpation of the praecordium revealed a prominent right ventricular heave, but the apex was undisplaced. Auscultation of the chest revealed scattered wheezes and coarse crepitations. Heart sounds were faint but normal.

These are the symptoms and signs of right heart failure and the most likely underlying cause in this man is chronic obstructive airways disease secondary to smoking. The systolic pulsations in the JVP are due to tricuspid regurgitation. As the right ventricle fails and dilates the tricuspid valve ring stretches and the valve may become incompetent.

Venous pressures on the right side of the heart increase as the right ventricle begins to fail. Any fall in right ventricular output also leads to a drop in output from the left heart as the left ventricle can only pump out what it has received from pulmonary venous return. Fluid retention in response to low cardiac output and high right-sided venous pressures causes congestion of the systemic veins. This disturbs the balance of hydrostatic and oncotic pressures leading to accumulation of fluid in the extravascular compartment. The main symptom of right heart failure is therefore ankle swelling. There may also be right upper quadrant discomfort due to hepatic congestion and abdominal swelling with ascites. Patients may get tired and breathless with exercise as left-sided output is limited by poor right ventricular function.

Clinical signs are due to venous congestion and include ankle oedema, a raised jugular venous pulse (JVP), a large palpable liver and sometimes ascites. Fluid may accumulate over the sacrum of patients confined to bed, giving rise to a sacral pad of oedema.

Sometimes the failing right ventricle becomes sufficiently dilated to stretch the tricuspid valve and cause it to become incompetent. During systole, therefore, blood regurgitates back into the right atrium. This may produce a pansystolic murmur over the tricuspid area and cause striking systolic pulsations in the neck and over the liver.

Acute on chronic heart failure

In most patients a combination of physiological adaptation and treatment leads to a steady (compensated) state where symptoms and signs are stable. Any abrupt deterioration from this compensated state is referred to as 'acute on chronic' heart failure and a cause should be sought. Paroxysmal arrhythmias (particularly tachyarrhythmias) are a common precipitant, as ventricular filling and coronary blood flow are both impaired at fast heart rates. Other precipitants of acute on chronic heart failure include poor compliance with treatment, myocardial infarction (sudden worsening heart failure is an important presentation of silent myocardial infarction), anaemia and infection.

INVESTIGATIONS

Heart failure is diagnosed mainly on clinical grounds but several investigations help confirm the diagnosis and elucidate an underlying cause. An ECG may show evidence of previous myocardial infarction or LV hypertrophy if heart failure is due to aortic stenosis or longstanding hypertension. There are no ECG features specific to dilated cardiomyopathy, although these patients frequently have conduction abnormalities (such as left bundle branch block) or non-specific T wave changes. A chest X-ray (CXR) may give some clues to the underlying cause (such as a large left atrium in mitral valve disease) but the following discussion deals only with the non-specific radiological features of heart failure.

Radiological features of heart failure

Heart size
With increased volumes of blood in the ventricles at the end of diastole these chambers gradually dilate. The size of the heart shadow on the CXR increases to greater than 50% of the thoracic diameter. This is called **cardiomegaly**.

Upper lobe blood diversion
The pattern of blood flow through the pulmonary circulation is not uniform due to the effects of gravity. At the lung apices venous and arterial pressures are lower than alveolar pressures. At the bases arterial and venous pressures are greater than intra-alveolar press-ures, so there is maximal pulmonary perfusion. Thus the venous pressure influences the degree of perfusion at various lung levels. In left heart failure pulmonary venous pressures are high. Blood is diverted from lower to upper zones in order to improve gas exchange. This is **upper lobe blood diversion** and causes a typical pattern of shadowing on the CXR, with prominent vascular markings in the upper zones. In severe left ventricular failure fluid collects in the alveolar spaces, causing typical opacities on the CXR. This alveolar shadowing often extends in a symmetrical pattern from the hila into the midzones giving rise to the so-called 'bats-wing' appearance of severe pulmonary oedema (Fig. 3.3).

Kerley's lines A and B
The bronchial tree and pulmonary vessels are supported by connective tissue. When pulmonary venous pressures are raised these tissues become thickened and oedematous, giving rise to characteristic shadows on the CXR. This is most marked at the lung bases producing short horizontal linear shadows. These are **Kerley B lines** and lie perpendicular to the pleural surface. **Kerley A lines** also occur with high pulmonary venous pressures but are less common. They are longer (up to 6 cm), are not restricted to the basal areas and do not extend to the pleural surface.

Pleural effusions
Fluid exchange across the capillary wall is governed by the balance of hydrostatic and oncotic forces (**Starling forces**). Movement out of a vessel is promoted by intravascular hydrostatic pressure and tissue oncotic pressure (the 'osmotic pull' provided by soluble proteins). Fluid resorption relies on tissue hydrostatic and intravascular oncotic pressures. With raised pulmonary venous pressures the balance of these forces is altered by the larger than normal intravascular hydrostatic pressure. Fluid accumulates in the extravascular compartment and seeps into the pleural space, giving rise to pleural effusions. The protein content of the fluid is low and is called a **transudate**. Protein-rich effusions that occur with intrathoracic malignancies and infections are termed **exudates**.

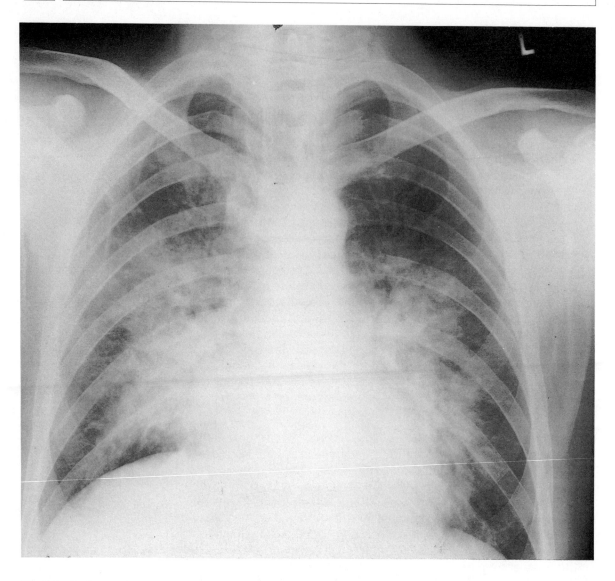

Fig. 3.3 Left ventricular failure. Note the typical perihilar 'batswing' shadowing.

Echocardiography

This is the most helpful investigation in determining the underlying cause of heart failure. Valvular causes are identified by their abnormal motion and by the presence of abnormal jets or pressures on Doppler studies. Lack of motion of a particular part of the myocardium suggests damage due to previous myocardial infarction. An increase in the dimensions of all the chambers suggests a dilated cardiomyopathy.

Case history
A 60-year-old woman saw her GP after returning from visiting her daughter and grandchildren during the school half term. She had noticed that her ankles had become swollen but attributed this to the hot weather. She had slept poorly while away and felt that the bed was too flat for her. Although active all her life she became short of breath when taking her grandchildren to the park. She denied chest pain or a cough. Examination revealed pitting oedema to the shins, venous pressure raised to 12 cm above the sternal angle, a slightly displaced apex beat but clear lung fields.

These are the classical symptoms of biventricular failure, namely ankle swelling, orthopnoea and exertional dyspnoea. She requires investigation with routine blood count, electrolytes, CXR and ECG. She should have an echocardiogram to look at ventricular size and function and to examine the cardiac valves. Once a precise diagnosis has been made appropriate treatment can be planned.

CAUSES OF HEART FAILURE

The list of causes of heart failure is long and only a few have been mentioned specifically in the text. It is useful and convenient to divide the list into easy to remember groups.

'Myocardial' causes of heart failure

This group includes **ischaemic heart disease** and **dilated cardiomyopathy**. Loss of myocardial function may happen suddenly in acute myocardial infarction, or take place over several years as a result of chronic ischaemia. Dilated cardiomyopathy is a disorder of unknown aetiology in which the left and/or right ventricle becomes dilated and functions very poorly (Fig. 3.4). Coronary anatomy is usually normal but the 'flabby' myocardium results in poor systolic emptying with symptoms and signs of heart failure.

Valvular causes of heart failure

Dysfunctioning valves place an extra haemodynamic burden on the heart. Regurgitation of left-sided valves (mitral and aortic) cause **volume overloading** of the left heart as the amount of blood in the ventricle at the end of diastole increases. Total stroke volume must increase in order to maintain useful cardiac output, as a significant proportion of the ejected blood is 'misdirected' (either back into the left atrium in mitral regurgitation, or back into the left ventricle in aortic regurgitation). Although not strictly 'valvular' it should be remembered that **congenital heart defects** (in particular **atrial and ventricular septal**

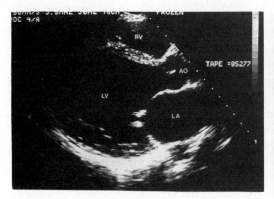 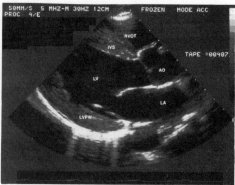

Fig. 3.4 Echocardiogram of a patient with a dilated, poorly contractile left ventricle alongside that of a normal patient for comparison.

defects) may cause heart failure, as part of the left ventricular output is misdirected into the pulmonary circulation through the septal defect. Congenital heart disorders are discussed more fully in Chapter 10.

'Afterload' causes of heart failure

High afterloads increase cardiac work as the myocardium must generate extra force to overcome the increased resistance to blood flow. A normally functioning ventricle is able to generate this extra force so that cardiac output is maintained and the system is said to be 'compensated'. If the extra burden persists over many years then the ability of the ventricle to overcome this resistance gradually declines, particularly if the afterload continues to increase. Cardiac output starts to fall and the system is said to 'decompensate'. The two major pathologies that increase the afterload on the left ventricle are **hypertension** and **aortic stenosis**.

Pericardial ('diastolic') causes of heart failure

Adequate diastolic filling of the ventricles is a prerequisite for a satisfactory cardiac output. If filling becomes impaired for any reason then cardiac output will fall. Restrictions of ventricular filling may occur if the pericardium itself is diseased (as in **constrictive pericarditis**) or if fluid (such as blood or malignant exudate) accumulates within the pericardium and the ventricle (called a **pericardial effusion**).

'Circulatory' causes of heart failure

Sometimes there is inadequate organ perfusion because the requirements of the peripheral tissues are abnormally high, rather than because of impaired cardiac output. Examples of conditions in which this may occur include **thyrotoxicosis** and severe **anaemia**. Cardiac output in these conditions is actually greater than normal, so it is probably better to regard them as conditions which may produce similar clinical features to heart failure rather than confuse them with specific cardiac abnormalities.

TREATMENT OF HEART FAILURE

Treatment of acute left ventricular failure

Acute LVF most commonly occurs as a result of myocardial infarction where an abrupt reduction in the pumping action of the heart causes a fall in cardiac output. Sympathetic-mediated vasoconstriction redirects blood centrally in an attempt to increase cardiac output along the Starling curve and maintain blood pressure. If the right ventricle is functioning normally then its output increases, but the dysfunctioning left ventricle is unable to increase its output. Fluid accumulates in the lungs and pulmonary oedema follows. Treatment of pulmonary oedema therefore involves measures that decrease right heart output or increase the output of the left heart, in addition to general supportive measures.

Patients with acute pulmonary oedema should be nursed sitting up with 60% oxygen delivered through a mask.

A reduction in venous tone may be achieved with intravenous **diamorphine**, which also alleviates the subjective sensation of breathlessness. It is a powerful **analgesic** so its use in the management of pulmonary oedema due to myocardial infarction is a logical one. It is generally given with a suitable anti-emetic such as **metoclopramide**.

Loop diuretics such as **frusemide**, given intravenously, act as venodilators long before any significant diuresis is seen. The subsequent diuretic action of frusemide helps reduce the volume overload of left ventricular failure. Intravenous or buccal GTN may also be useful. Acute LVF not due to infarction may be either valvular in origin or, more commonly, occurs when the balance of chronic compensated left heart failure is upset by, for example, an arrhythmia or non-compliance with treatment. The most common rhythm disturbance to precipitate

---

Treatment of acute LVF 'at a glance'

1. Sit up
2. 60% oxygen
3. IV access
4. IV opiates with anti-emetic
5. IV diuretic
6. Nitrates (iv or buccal)
7. Consider, where appropriate, digoxin, inotropic support, invasive monitoring, ventilatory assistance, balloon pump.

acute on chronic heart failure is **atrial fibrillation. Digoxin** is the drug of choice in this situation.

Treatment of chronic left ventricular failure

Most chronic left ventricular failure is due either to chronic ischaemia or hypertension. Until comparatively recently the treatment of chronic left ventricular failure was aimed mainly at relieving symptoms, but the advent of angiotensin converting enzyme inhibitors has also improved long-term survival in these patients.

There are three broad strategies that may be employed in the treatment of chronic left heart failure, which may be understood with the aid of Fig. 3.5.

Diuretics and nitrates ('venous' drugs)

Drugs which reduce fluid overload are useful in relieving the symptoms of chronic left ventricular failure. **Diuretics**, together with sensible restrictions in the intake of dietary sodium, help to reduce central venous pressures. Since the ventricular function curve is virtually flat there is little fall in cardiac output as a result of this reduction in preload. For most patients with mild heart failure a **thiazide** diuretic such as **bendrofluazide** is adequate to return central venous pressures towards normal and relieve symptoms. Their adverse effects on glucose and lipid metabolism are unlikely to be a significant problem in the elderly but make them slightly less desirable for long-term use in younger patients. If the disease progresses, or if symptoms are not adequately controlled with a thiazide, then a more powerful **loop diuretic** such as **frusemide** may be required.

If diuretics are not sufficient to off-load the congested venous system then drugs that dilate the venous vascular bed may be added. Hence, **nitrates** such as **isosorbide mononitrate** are commonly used for symptomatic relief in chronic left ventricular failure. Although nitrates and

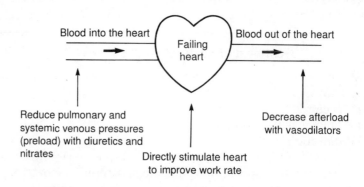

Fig. 3.5 Strategies for treating heart failure.

diuretics give haemodynamically satisfying results in that they reduce central venous pressures towards normal, it has yet to be shown conclusively that they have any effect on long-term survival in heart failure.

Diuretic therapy

Diuretics are drugs which act on the kidneys to increase sodium and water excretion. They are classified mainly on their site of action on the renal tubules, as shown in Fig. 3.6.

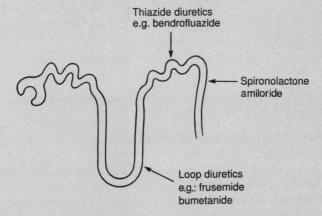

Fig. 3.6   Sites of action of various diuretics in the renal tubule.

Loop diuretics
These inhibit active transport of sodium from the ascending limb of the loop of Henle, thereby reducing the concentrating power of the kidneys. The large load of sodium remaining in the distal tubule cannot be completely reabsorbed, so that sodium (and therefore water) is lost in the urine. The increased amount of sodium present in the distal tubule leads to increased exchange of sodium for potassium or hydrogen, which may cause hypokalaemia and alkalosis. Patients treated with frusemide or bumetanide should have their potassium monitored closely for the first few weeks of therapy. If the potassium falls a potassium-sparing diuretic (such as amiloride) should be added. Long-term therapy with loop diuretics may lead, particularly in the elderly, to dehydration and profound electrolyte depletion.

Thiazides
These inhibit the transport of sodium and chloride in the proximal part of the distal tubule. The increased availability of sodium for exchange in the distal tubule may, like loop diuretics, lead to

potassium loss. Other important side-effects of thiazide diuretics include hyperuricaemia (occasionally causing gout), hyperglycaemia and hyperlipidaemia.

Potassium-sparing diuretics
These inhibit the sodium for potassium/hydrogen exchange mechanism in the distal part of the distal tubule. This ion exchanger is under the control of the hormone **aldosterone**. **Spironolactone** is a direct antagonist of aldosterone and inhibits the effect of the high levels of this hormone that occur in heart failure (secondary hyperaldosteronism). Amiloride, by a different mechanism, also inhibits this exchanger. Potassium-sparing diuretics help prevent electrolyte disturbances caused by loop and thiazide diuretics.

Angiotensin-converting enzyme inhibitors (arterial and venous vasodilators)

Drugs such as **captopril** and **enalapril** have been shown to improve long-term survival in patients with congestive cardiac failure. The inhibition of angiotensin-converting enzyme (ACE) results in decreased circulating levels of the vasoconstrictor angiotensin II. This reduces both **venous and arterial** vascular tone, thereby improving the pre- and afterload demands placed on the heart. Damping down of the angiotensin–aldosterone axis also reduces the avid (and inappropriate) salt and water retention that occurs in cardiac failure in response to poor renal perfusion.

When starting treatment with ACE inhibitors for heart failure it is generally advised that patients are in bed, as profound hypotension and even acute renal failure are occasional first-dose complications. This is because glomerular filtration relies on the head of pressure created by the tone of the afferent and efferent arterioles on either side of the glomerulus. Angiotensin acts on both of these vessels, but does so to a greater extent on the smooth muscle of the **efferent** arteriole. Loss of tone in the efferent arteriole reduces pressure in the glomerulus. If the reduction is excessive then acute renal failure may follow, although this is uncommon.

Some fall off in glomerular filtration rate (GFR) is usually seen with ACE inhibitors and it is probably this that accounts for the variable degree of potassium retention that accompanies use of these drugs. It is usual practice to stop other potassiuim-retaining drugs such as amiloride when starting treatment with ACE inhibitors.

Case history

A 64-year-old man was brought to hospital by ambulance with acute breathlessness. He often woke at night feeling the need for fresh air but on this occasion awoke sweating, with palpitations and fighting for air. On examination in Casualty he was sweating profusely with cold peripheries. His respiratory rate was 50/min and he had a weak, thready chaotic pulse of 140/min. Auscultation revealed a gallop rhythm and fine crepitations to the mid–zones bilaterally.

This man is in pulmonary oedema which is a medical emergency. He should be sat up, given 60% oxygen by face mask and attached to a cardiac monitor. Intravenous access must be established immediately and he should be given intravenous diamorphine and an anti-emetic. Once the opiates have helped relieve the sensation of acute suffocation he should be given intravenous diuretic to reduce pulmonary venous pressure.

Further history revealed that he had suffered from exertional dyspnoea and 3 pillow orthopnoea for several months. Investigations had shown a dilated poorly contractile left ventricle and he was treated with diuretics and ACE inhibitors. The acute deterioration was due in this case to the onset of atrial fibrillation as the impairment of diastolic filling and the reduction in coronary blood flow precipitated pulmonary oedema. Echocardiography showed a dilated left atrium and no attempt was made at cardioversion. He was given digoxin to control the ventricular rate and warfarin to reduce the risk of systemic embolism.

Direct stimulation of the failing heart (inotropes)

Digoxin is particularly useful if heart failure is precipitated or made worse by the onset of atrial fibrillation (AF). If the ventricular response rate is rapid then the symptoms of heart failure will be worsened for two reasons. First, tachycardia and loss of co-ordinated atrial systole impair diastolic filling so cardiac output falls. Second, coronary blood flow becomes impaired at fast rates as the heart spends less time in diastole. Oxygen delivery is impaired which depresses cardiac performance still further.

The use of digoxin for patients in sinus rhythm is controversial. It is a weak positive inotrope and studies show that some patients in sinus rhythm may benefit. Most people reserve digoxin for patients in AF or in those whose symptoms do not respond to diuretics and ACE inhibitors.

CARDIOGENIC SHOCK

Shock is a rather non-specific term used to describe the condition in which hypotension results in poor blood flow to all the tissues of the body. Cardiogenic shock refers to catastrophic circulatory collapse due to a primary cardiac cause. It is usually the result of **massive myocardial infarction**, where the amount of contractile muscle is suddenly reduced.

Monitoring of patients in shock

Successful treatment of shock depends on careful measurement and monitoring of the important indices of cardiovascular function, so that the appropriate haemodynamic support may be provided. These indices include pulse, blood pressure, central venous pressure and urine output. If the shock has a circulatory or haemorrhagic cause then central venous pressure gives an adequate guide to the filling pressures of both sides of the heart. However, in cardiogenic shock there is a disparity in function between the two ventricles. Most cases of cardiogenic shock are due to LV dysfunction and its function curve is much flatter than that of the right, as shown in Fig. 3.7.

Given that stroke volume of the two ventricles is the same, then from the diagram it can be seen that, for any given cardiac output, left-sided filling pressures must be greater than those on the right. Under such circumstances, measurements of central venous pressure become meaningless and a method is required for determining left ventricular filling pressures. This is achieved, indirectly, by measuring pressures in the pulmonary arterial system with a **Swan Ganz catheter**. A catheter with a balloon mounted at its tip is introduced via a large vein into the right atrium. Following its inflation the balloon is floated through the right side of the heart and into the pulmonary trunk until it will pass no further. At this point there is a continuous column of fluid between the distal lumen of the catheter and the left atrium because there are no intervening valves. The pressure at this point is recorded and is called the pulmonary capillary wedge pressure (PCWP). It reflects the pressure in the pulmonary venous system and is, therefore, an **indirect** measure of left atrial filling pressure.

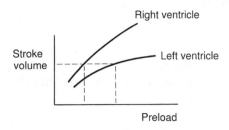

Fig. 3.7 Right and left ventricular function curves in cardiogenic shock.

Cardiogenic shock in context

The term 'shock' describes a clinical syndrome in which poor organ perfusion gives rise to cool peripheries, oliguria and cerebral dysfunction. There are many causes of shock, but a useful way of grouping and understanding them is to think of poor perfusion as having either a central (cardiac) or a peripheral (vascular) cause. In the first group the heart, for some reason, is unable to pump blood effectively. In the second there is normal (or even increased) cardiac output but some 'disturbance' of the vascular tree (either involving circulating volume or a very low peripheral resistance) causes blood pressure to fall.

Central (cardiac) causes

Cardiogenic shock has already been mentioned and describes the syndrome of hypotension and poor peripheral perfusion secondary to poor cardiac output. Most commonly it occurs following massive **myocardial infarction** where the remaining viable myocardium is unable to maintain the circulation. Another cause of cardiogenic shock is acute mitral regurgitation. Blood is misdirected back into the LA, rather than forward into the circulation, so that cardiac output and blood pressure both fall. This often causes acute pulmonary oedema and, rapidly, death.

In **'obstructive' cardiac shock** the myocardium itself contracts normally but its action is somehow constrained. In **massive pulmonary embolism** the outflow of the right ventricle is obstructed by the presence of a large occluding thrombus in one of the major pulmonary arteries. Given that left ventricular output is dependent on venous return from the pulmonary circulation, cardiac output into the systemic circulation falls dramatically despite a normally contractile left heart.

Left ventricular output may also be restricted by the prevention of efficient diastolic filling. The presence of fluid (usually either blood or malignant exudate) within the pericardium (**pericardial effusion**) may limit ventricular filling (and therefore output) sufficiently to cause the syndrome of shock. This is termed **cardiac tamponade**.

'Peripheral' (circulatory) causes

Here, in spite of a normal or even increased cardiac output some 'abnormality' of the vascular tree causes hypotension and the syndrome of shock. Two distinct groups are recognized: those where the circulating volume is normal and those where it is low.

Normovolaemia
The classic example of normovolaemic non-cardiac shock is **sepsis**. Endotoxins released by bacteria cause arteriolar vasodilatation so that peripheral resistance is inappropriately low. The heart beats faster and more strongly but is still unable to maintain blood pressure.

Hypovolaemia
Massive blood loss may eventually lead to shock. Blood loss may be obvious (revealed) such as haematemesis from an upper gastrointestinal bleed; or concealed (such as a leaking aortic aneurysm where blood is lost into the peritoneal cavity).

In a few patients cardiogenic shock is due to severe right ventricular damage. Such patients become hypotensive because the right ventricle is unable to drive blood through the pulmonary circulation. Pulmonary venous return is therefore low so left-sided cardiac output is inadequate.

Peripheral causes of shock (either vasodilatation or blood loss) are associated with lower than normal wedge pressures. In cardiogenic shock poor ventricular emptying leads to high left ventricular end diastolic pressures. Pulmonary venous pressures rise and high pulmonary capillary wedge pressures are recorded.

Treatment of cardiogenic shock

The vaso-constriction that occurs in cardiogenic shock increases afterload on an already dysfunctioning left ventricle. The aim of treatment in cardiogenic shock is to optimize the loads against which the ventricle must work, thereby increasing cardiac output and improving the symptoms of poor perfusion. Vasodilators such as intravenous glyceryl trinitrate (GTN) or sodium nitroprusside are most commonly used for this purpose. GTN is mainly a venous dilator, whereas nitroprusside also dilates arterioles, thereby reducing afterload. Both decrease venous return and therefore left atrial pressures which helps pulmonary congestion. Better systolic emptying also helps reduce left ventricular end diastolic pressures. Care must be taken not to induce hypotension, as the resultant reflex tachycardia may increase myocardial oxygen requirements.

Inotropes

These are drugs that act directly on ß-1 receptors in myocardial tissue to increase the amount of work done by the heart. All, however, increase myocardial demand for oxygen. It is thought that, by increasing oxygen consumption, inotropes may in fact extend the ischaemic areas or even precipitate infarction in those areas of myocardium that are already critically ischaemic. Hence the choice of inotrope must be a careful one.

Dopamine is a naturally occurring catecholamine that has both α-and β-adrenergic effects. In addition to its positive effects on heart rate and stroke volume, dopamine has other important actions. At low doses it causes dilatation of skeletal and splanchnic arterioles, thereby reducing peripheral resistance. This vasodilator effect is also seen in the kidney where dopamine increases renal perfusion and improves urine output.

At higher doses, the α-effects of dopamine predominate and peripheral vasoconstriction is the dominant feature. This vasoconstriction increases venous return and ventricular filling pressure; a dangerous effect if left-sided pressures are already high, secondary to poor systolic emptying. Higher doses of dopamine also cause release of noradrenaline

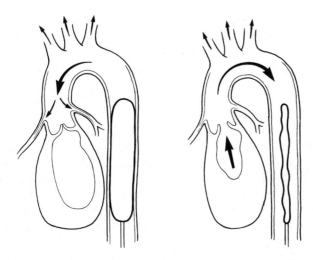

Fig. 3.8 Balloon counterpulsation. During diastole the balloon inflates and pressure increases in the proximal aorta which aids coronary perfusion. The balloon deflates during systole, decreasing afterload.

from the adrenal medulla which in turn, via their α-adrenergic action, mediate arteriolar vasoconstriction and increase peripheral resistance. The vasoconstrictive effects of high-dose dopamine may be offset by the use of vasodilators such as sodium nitroprusside.

Dobutamine is closely related to dopamine and was synthesized in an attempt to separate the inotropic and chronotropic properties of β-agonists, since tachycardia increases myocardial oxygen consumption. It has a powerful positive inotropic effect when given intravenously to patients with heart failure, but with less effect on heart rate. No specific effect is seen on the renal vasculature, but urine output improves as cardiac output increases. For a given increase in oxygen requirement, dobutamine leads to more improvement in cardiac output than dopamine.

Balloon counterpulsation

This is a method of providing temporary mechanical assistance to a failing left ventricle. A balloon of approximately 40 cm^3 capacity is passed via the femoral artery to lie in the thoracic aorta just below the aortic arch (Fig. 3.8). It is triggered from the ECG to inflate immediately after closure of the aortic valve and deflate just prior to the onset of ventricular systole. The presence of the inflated balloon in diastole augments aortic diastolic pressure, thereby aiding coronary and cerebral perfusion. Deflation of the balloon in systole reduces the afterload on the left ventricle and favours flow of blood forward into the circulation. Balloon counterpulsation is suitable only in situations where there is a potentially remediable cause of the failing ventricle such as acute mitral regurgitation or ventricular septal defect following myocardial infarction. It is also used in unstable angina to augment coronary blood flow and should, in such circumstances be followed by early angiography and intervention, either with angioplasty or surgery.

Prognosis

Even with the benefit of intensive monitoring and haemodynamic support the prognosis of cardiogenic shock due to 'pump failure' is grave. A downward spiral is established in which arterial hypotension from pump dysfunction causes a reduction in coronary blood flow and poor coronary perfusion further impairs pump function. Relatives should be informed of the extent of the damage to the heart and that the outlook may be poor.

Ischaemic heart disease $\boxed{4}$

PHYSIOLOGICAL BACKGROUND

The rate of myocardial oxygen consumption is determined by a combination of the heart rate, the force of ventricular contraction, the volume of blood in the ventricles at the end of diastolic filling and the resistance against which the ventricles must contract. In order to function efficiently, heart muscle (myocardium) requires an adequate flow of oxygenated blood via the coronary arteries. Blood flow through a vessel depends partly on the diameter of that vessel and partly on the head of pressure driving the blood through. Hence reductions in myocardial blood supply may occur when coronary arteries become narrowed.

ISCHAEMIA

This term describes the condition in which there is a mismatch in the cell between oxygen demand and supply. A generalized disorder of metabolism results in which anaerobic glycolysis produces lactic acid, causing a lowered intracellular pH and impaired contractile function of heart muscle.

ANGINA

Angina is the clinical correlate of myocardial ischaemia and is the term used to describe the pain or discomfort that occurs when the oxygen demand of the heart exceeds its supply (Fig. 4.1). It is a simple concept and says nothing about the underlying cause of the impaired supply. Patients may use a variety of words to describe the symptoms of angina, including 'tightness', 'pressing', 'choking', 'constricting', 'like a tight band' or as though 'someone is sitting on my chest'. Many dismiss their symptoms as being due to 'indigestion'. Classically the pain is felt **retro-sternally** but may also radiate to the arms, back, neck or jaw and, indeed, may be felt in one of these sites only. Generally the pain is precipitated by physical, emotional or mental stress and dies away when the original trigger is removed. In most patients it is relieved by sublingual **glyceryl trinitrate** (**GTN**) tablets or spray and in the context of General Practice this may be a valuable diagnostic test.

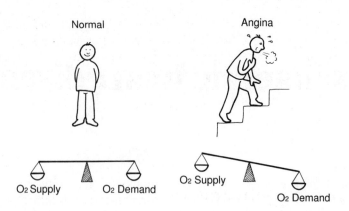

Fig. 4.1 Cartoon representation of angina. (a) Oxygen supply is equal to demand and the man is asymptomatic. In (b) exercise outstrips the available supply of oxygen and the man develops chest pain.

Precipitants of angina

Exercise is the most frequent precipitant of angina as the associated tachycardia, increased force of contraction and greater preload all increase oxygen consumption. Other important precipitants include **emotion** and **eating** which increase sympathetic stimulation of the heart. Heart rate and the force of myocardial contraction both rise and oxygen consumption is increased as the amount of 'work' the heart must do increases. Another common precipitant is **cold weather**. Peripheral vasoconstriction leads to greater central pooling of blood with a rise in ventricular load and oxygen demand. In addition cold air may cause coronary vasoconstriction, which reduces coronary blood flow.

Precipitants of angina

Exercise
Eating
Cold weather
Emotional stress

Patterns of angina

Many patients who experience the symptoms of angina do so after a predictable and reproducible level of activity and are described as having **chronic stable angina** or **angina of effort**. It should be stressed that severity of symptoms and the amount of exercise required to precipitate them correlate poorly with the extent of underlying coronary artery disease.

Patients who experience angina at rest or who have rapidly worsening angina are said to have **unstable angina**. This is very serious since it may be the prelude to death (infarction) of myocardial tissue and is therefore sometimes termed **pre-infarction** or **crescendo** angina. The symptoms of unstable angina are similar to those of angina of effort but, typically, the pain is more severe, lasts longer and is less well relieved by sublingual nitrates. The diagnosis is based chiefly on the history and typical ECG findings and is discussed more fully below.

MYOCARDIAL INFARCTION

This term refers to death of heart muscle, usually as a result of prolonged ischaemia. The resultant pain is continuous and generally more severe than that of angina of effort. The myocardium affected by infarction never recovers and heals by fibrosis. Myocardial infarction and its distinction from unstable angina is dealt with more extensively later in this chapter.

In most patients angina is due to obstruction of coronary arteries as a consequence of **atherosclerosis**, but may also occur in patients with normal coronary arteries. For example in **aortic stenosis** the left ventricle undergoes hypertrophy in order to generate sufficient force to overcome the obstruction to its outlet and drive blood into the aorta. This increases myocardial oxygen demand which is not met by the existing coronary circulation.

Structure of a normal artery (Fig. 4.2)

The **intima** begins with the endothelium and underneath this lie smooth muscle cells in an extracellular matrix. The **media** is bounded by the internal and external lamina and consists of variable amounts of elastic tissue and smooth muscle cells. Large elastic vessels such as the aorta contain much more elastin than smaller muscular arteries. **The adventitia**, the outermost layer, consists mainly of connective tissue and small blood vessels.

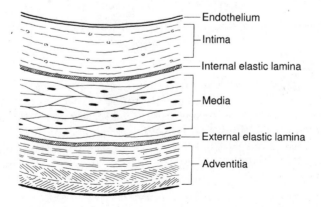

— Endothelium

— Intima

— Internal elastic lamina

— Media

— External elastic lamina

— Adventitia

Fig. 4.2 Schematic diagram of a normal artery.

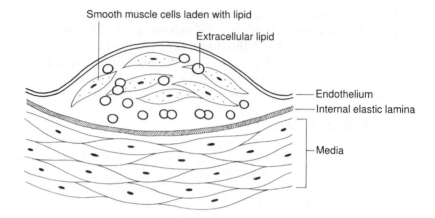

Fig. 4.3 Schematic diagram of an atheromatous plaque. The media contains abundant intra- and extracellular lipid.

Why do coronary arteries become narrowed?

Ischaemic heart disease usually occurs as a consequence of **atherosclerosis**. This is a disease of large and medium-sized arteries, in which the arterial lumen becomes progressively narrowed by the growth of fibro-fatty lesions called atheromatous **plaques** (Fig. 4.3).

The lesion
The basic lesion of atherosclerosis is the **fibrous plaque**, which has three components. The **cellular** component consists of smooth muscle cells and macrophages. Collagen and elastin form the **connective tissue** element and there may be an abundance of intra and extracellular **lipid**.

Risk factors for atherosclerosis

There are several risk factors that predispose to this disease, which include:

Age and gender
Atherosclerosis is strongly correlated with age and sex. Whether age itself is a risk factor or merely reflects length of exposure to other risk factors is not clear, but the incidence of atherosclerotic lesions increases steadily after the third decade and is more common in males than females during these years. Following the menopause atherosclerosis accelerates in women, so that by the age of 70 there is little difference between the sexes. HRT reduces the risk of ischaemic heart disease (IHD) in post-menopausal women.

Smoking

The exact percentage increased risk is not known, but most people believe that smokers are at least twice as likely to die from coronary artery disease as non-smokers. Ex-smokers gradually assume the normal risk pattern and return to normal after about 10 years.

Genetics

There is no doubt that ischaemic heart disease runs in families. Some of this may be as a result of other risk factors being inherited but there is an additional latent factor, as there are families with high rates of ischaemic heart disease where none of the other risk factors are present. Ischaemic heart disease is more common among certain racial groups (such as those from the Indian subcontinent), which also suggests a 'genetic predisposition'.

Lipids

There is overwhelming evidence to suggest that having high blood lipid levels (in particular **hypercholesterolaemia**) is an important risk factor for the development of atherosclerosis. Certain genetic disorders (most notably familial hypercholesterolaemia) are associated with premature death from myocardial infarction despite the absence of any other risk factors for atherosclerosis. Over 70% of total plasma cholesterol is in the form of low density lipoproteins (LDLs) and it is with high levels of this type of lipoprotein that the development of atherosclerosis is most closely correlated.

Diabetes mellitus

Both insulin and non-insulin dependent diabetes mellitus increase the risk of developing coronary artery disease. Good glycaemic control is important in reducing the likelihood of developing all forms of vascular disease but does not completely abolish the risk.

Hypertension

This is an important risk factor for coronary disease and seems to be particularly important in the presence of other risk factors. It is not clear if control of hypertension reduces the risk of developing ischaemic heart disease, although it certainly reduces the risk of stroke.

Although the risk factors for IHD and the histological appearance of the atherosclerotic plaques are all well studied, the pathogenesis of these lesions is still largely unresolved.

Reaction to injury hypothesis

This hypothesis incites some form of **endothelial injury** as the primary event in initiating atherosclerosis (Fig. 4.4). The word

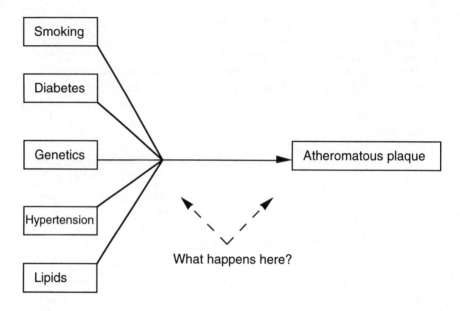

Fig. 4.4 Risk factors for ischaemic heart disease.

'injury' here includes physical (i.e. mechanical) damage; chemical insult, such as abnormal circulating levels of lipoproteins and cholesterol; and electrical abnormalities such as the abnormal glycosylation of surface proteins and carbohydrates that occurs in diabetes. These various insults create a **dysfunctioning endothelium**; one whose cell junctions have been breached to expose subendothelial collagen and one whose permeability to lipid is abnormally high. The presence of cholesterol in the sub-endothelial tissues also stimulates the reactionary processes described below.

Whatever the damage or insult, platelets adhere to the abnormal endothelial surface and release a variety of growth factors and cytokines akin to those involved in wound healing. Smooth muscle cells from the media migrate in response to the stimuli and begin to synthesize extracellular matrix. Macrophages and smooth muscle cells become laden with lipid, which is also deposited extracellularly.

INVESTIGATIONS

In patients with suspected coronary artery disease, investigations are aimed at establishing the severity and extent of disease; and at identifying potentially reversible risk factors such as hypercholesterolaemia. The resting ECG is frequently normal, but the presence of pathological Q waves suggests previous infarction. A widely used non-invasive investigation is the **exercise test**, described in Chapter 2. It is used in several contexts and the diagnostic information should always be interpreted in the light of the clinical setting. In middle aged or elderly patients a typical history of angina is almost certainly due to coronary disease and in such patients the exercise test serves to give an idea of the extent of disease. S–T segment changes at a low workload or a fall in blood pressure with exercise are indicators of severe disease and angiography should be considered. Young patients with an atypical history are less likely to have significant coronary artery disease and a positive exercise test in these patients may not represent underlying ischaemia (the so-called false-positive test). Between these two extremes lie many patients with a moderate probability of significant coronary disease. In these patients the exercise test is a valuable method of acquiring evidence to confirm or refute the diagnosis and plan management.

There are several situations in which **coronary angiography** is performed. These include young patients who have had a myocardial infarction or who have a typical history of angina; recurrent angina following myocardial infarction; angina that cannot be controlled medically; patients with unstable angina; and patients with very abnormal exercise tests suggestive of extensive disease.

TREATMENT OF CHRONIC STABLE ANGINA

Treatment is aimed at minimizing the risk of developing further atheromatous disease and prompt attention to the consequences of IHD (notably angina and infarction, but also cardiac failure and arrhythmias).

Chest pain is frightening and some patients believe that they are having a 'heart attack' each time they experience pain. Patients with angina therefore require careful explanation of the cause of their pain. Many benefit symptomatically from reassurance, explanation and advice about exercising within their own pain limit. Patients should be encouraged to become 'acquainted' with their angina and to report any changes in its pattern. Further treatment may be divided into general measures, drug therapy and procedures on the coronary arteries aimed at restoring an adequate myocardial blood supply.

General measures

These include, where relevant, stopping smoking, regular gentle exercise, dietary advice, weight reduction and control of blood pressure. **Drug therapy** aims to adjust the balance of oxygen supply and demand, so that coronary blood flow is adequate despite persistent arterial stenosis. In addition low dose **aspirin** (75–150 mg daily) inhibits platelet aggregation and reduces the likelihood of intracoronary thrombosis.

Nitrates

Nitrates act by relaxing vascular smooth muscle in systemic and coronary arteries and veins. This systemic vasodilator activity decreases myocardial oxygen demand by reducing both preload (venous pressure and therefore intraventricular end diastolic pressure are lowered) and afterload (by lowering blood pressure). Dilatation of the coronary vessels also improves coronary perfusion. Most episodes of angina are relieved within 2–3 minutes by sublingual glyceryl trinitrate (GTN), either in tablet or aerosol form. Patients should be advised to spit out or swallow GTN tablets once the pain has resolved to avoid the pounding headache that often accompanies GTN usage. Taking a tablet before exercise is a useful prophylactic manoeuvre.

Patients who experience angina regularly or after only moderate exertion require regular prophylaxis. Options include longer-acting, slow-release nitrates, β-blockers and calcium antagonists. Oral **isosorbide dinitrate**, or its active metabolite **isosorbide mononitrate**, provide similar, longer lasting, activity to GTN.

Beta-adrenoceptor antagonists (ß-blockers)

β-Blockers are effective prophylactic agents against angina and are particularly appropriate if there is co-existent hypertension. They slow the heart rate and reduce the force of myocardial contraction, both of which lower myocardial oxygen demand. **Propranolol** is a widely used β-blocker, but is non-selective and acts not only on cardiac (β-1), but also on β-2 receptors in the peripheral tissues. Hence, adverse effects such as tiredness, broncho-constriction and prolonged recovery from diabetic hypoglycaemia are more frequent. **Atenolol** and **metoprolol** are more cardio-selective in their actions. Care should be taken in withdrawing β-blockers after more than a few weeks of treatment as worsening angina and even myocardial infarction may rarely be precipitated.

Calcium antagonists

These include **nifedipine**, **verapamil**, **diltiazem** and **amlodipine** all of which inhibit the transmembrane influx of calcium and impair intracellular activation mechanisms. Their use in the relief of angina relates to a variable mixture of a lowering of the contractile state of the myocardium, a reduction in vascular resistance (which reduces afterload) and coronary artery vasodilatation. Choice of calcium antagonist may be influenced by co-existent disease and treatment. Nifedipine acts predominantly on vascular smooth muscle cells. The vasodilatation induced by nifedipine may, via the baroreceptor mechanism, mediate a **reflex tachycardia**. This increases myocardial demand for oxygen and may worsen angina if used alone. When given for angina nifedipine is best used in combination with a β-blocker. Verapamil and diltiazem lower heart rate by their actions on the pacemaking SA node and AV nodal conduction. Side-effects of calcium channel blockers are due to vasodilatation and include **headache**, **flushing**, **dizziness** and (particularly with nifedipine) **ankle oedema**.

Drug treatment of chronic stable angina

Aspirin
Nitrate spray/tablets to use when symptoms occur
β-blockers (if no contraindication)
Calcium antagonists
Long-acting nitrates

Interventions aimed at restoring coronary blood flow

Some patients require consideration for revascularization. This requires a knowledge of the anatomy of the diseased coronary circulation which is achieved with coronary angiography. In this technique (described in detail in Chapter 2), X-ray pictures are taken following the injection of radio-opaque dye into the coronary circulation. Once the lesion or lesions have been identified with angiography the appropriate revascularization procedure can be planned. One option is to relieve the coronary obstruction by dilatation with a balloon (percutaneous transluminal coronary **angioplasty [PTCA]**). An alternative, more invasive, procedure is to bypass the obstruction **surgically**.

Surgical treatment of ischaemic heart disease

With this form of treatment about 80% of patients enjoy complete symptom relief, with partial relief in a further 10–15%. The aim of surgery is to bypass the stenosis or stenoses using one of the following techniques:

Coronary artery vein bypass grafting

This involves the use of the patient's own saphenous vein to bypass the obstruction (Fig. 4.5). The heart is rendered motionless either by ischaemic arrest or with cold concentrated potassium solution. The original distal end of the vein is made proximal (i.e. nearest to aorta) so that the natural direction of the venous valves favours coronary blood flow. There is little increase in morbidity with increasing number of grafts, so the aim is to bypass all stenoses.

Internal mammary artery grafting

Here the patient's internal mammary artery is mobilized and grafted onto a coronary artery distal to the obstruction. Being a vessel designed for

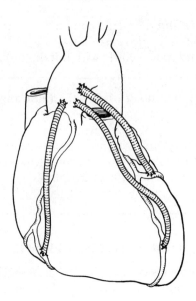

Fig. 4.5   Coronary artery bypass grafting.

high pressures it has a lower occlusion rate than vein grafting. Anatomical problems limit the use of this excellent graft to lesions in the arteries at the front of the heart (i.e. in the left anterior descending artery).

Angioplasty

Percutaneous transluminal coronary angioplasty (PTCA) is used in the treatment of selected patients with angina. A guiding catheter is introduced into the femoral artery and passed via the aorta into the mouth of the coronary artery. A guide wire is then passed through the catheter and manipulated into the artery with the stenosis to be treated. An inflatable balloon mounted on a thin catheter is then passed across the stenosis in the deflated state using X-ray screening. The balloon is then inflated to dilate the artery and relieve the obstruction (Fig. 4.6). It was previously used mainly for patients with isolated, proximal, non-calcified atheromatous lesions. More recently, however, an increasing number of patients with multi-vessel disease have been treated successfully with angioplasty. The main limitation with this technique is that the artery at the site of dilatation may re-narrow, usually within six months of the procedure. This causes recurrence of symptoms in about 25% of patients, when either further PTCA or bypass surgery may be offered.

Coronary artery stenting

Stents are tubular mesh-like structures made of metal. In the collapsed state they are sufficiently narrow to be passed into coronary arteries on

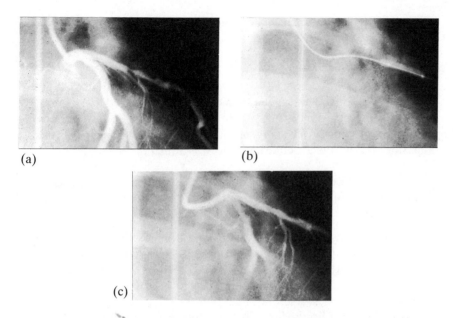

(a)

(b)

(c)

Fig. 4.6 Percutaneous transluminal coronary angioplasty (PTCA). Angiography outlines the coronary anatomy (a) A balloon is passed across the stenosis and inflated (b) to improve the patency of the vessel (c).

an angioplasty balloon. The balloon is then inflated and the expanded stent remains to 'scaffold' the coronary artery and help maintain lumen patency. Stents may be used as an emergency procedure if coronary artery dissection complicates angioplasty. The stent supports the dissection flap and prevents it from occluding the lumen. It is likely that stents will be used more widely as recent evidence suggests that the restenosis rate is less than for simple angioplasty. Most patients require the anti-platelet drug **ticlopidine** in addition to aspirin following stent insertion for one month in order to minimize the risk of stent thrombosis.

Other techniques

There exist several other techniques aimed at improving coronary blood flow. **Laser therapy** aims to 'burn away' atheromatous plaques. **Directional coronary atherectomy** uses a device that cuts sideways into the lesion and removes slices of atheroma which are stored in the tip of the catheter and subsequently removed. A **coronary artery rotablator** aims to abrade atheroma by use of a rotating burr. The use of these techniques in clinical practice is limited, particularly as they do not reduce the restenosis rate.

Case history

A 45-year-old man consulted his GP because he had been experiencing mild chest tightness when playing football with his 7-year-old son. He was a heavy smoker of 25 years and had a strong family history of coronary artery disease, his father and two brothers having suffered myocardial infarctions in their early fifties. Examination was unremarkable, as was a resting 12-lead ECG.

This man describes a classical history of angina and should be investigated further. **Management** therefore involves the following:

- Careful explanation of the cause of his symptoms so that he understands the need for steps to modify his risk factors. At this stage there is no need to inform the DVLA unless angina is precipitated by driving. (N.B. The DVLA must be informed if HGV/PSV drivers develop angina.)
- Attention to risk factors. He should be advised strongly to stop smoking. His lipids should be checked and, if elevated, he should receive appropriate dietary advice. Lipid lowering therapy may also be considered.
- He should be started on regular aspirin and given GTN spray to use when symptoms occur. Regular follow-up will be needed in order to monitor his symptoms and adjust therapy as required.
- He requires urgent hospital referral to a cardiologist for consideration of angiography. An exercise test may be helpful to give some idea as to the urgency with which this should be undertaken. In the meantime he should be told to seek urgent medical attention if his angina worsens or he develops symptoms at rest.

UNSTABLE ANGINA

If symptoms of angina occur at rest or are rapidly worsening the term unstable angina is used. It frequently heralds myocardial infarction, so is also termed 'pre-infarction' or 'crescendo' angina. The pain of unstable angina is similar to that of chronic stable angina but is characteristically more intense, lasts longer and is less well relieved by sublingual nitrates. Unstable angina may be the first presentation of ischaemic heart disease or occur as an abrupt change in an established pattern of angina of effort.

The diagnosis of unstable angina is based chiefly on the history but is aided by the presence of minor, usually reversible, changes in the ECG that reflect underlying ischaemia. These include **lowering of the S–T segments** and **T wave inversion** in the leads that examine the area of ischaemic myocardium (Fig. 4.7). It must be remembered that the absence of ECG changes does not exclude the diagnosis of unstable angina.

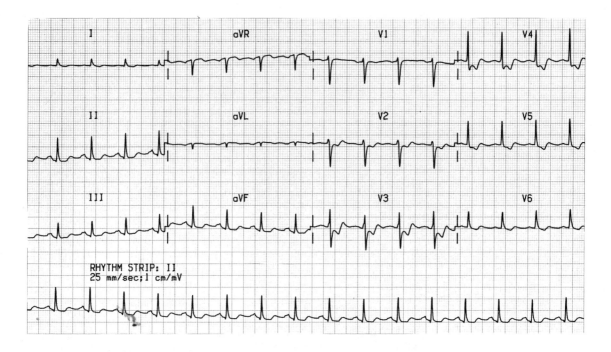

Fig. 4.7   ECG of a patient with unstable angina. Note the S–T depression in leads I, aVL and V_{2-6}.

Chest pain initially thought to be unstable angina may, in fact, originate from evolving myocardial infarction. Serial cardiac enzyme levels provide the best evidence (albeit retrospective) for myocardial infarction and should always be carried out in patients with unstable angina.

Treatment of unstable angina

Unstable angina is a medical emergency. Untreated, 30% of all patients with unstable angina will either have died or suffered myocardial infarction within three months. Patients are best managed in specialized **Coronary Care Units (CCUs)** where arrhythmias and progressive ECG changes can be monitored. The aims of management of unstable angina are to relieve the acute pain of ischaemia, to prevent recurrence of that ischaemia and establish a new, more stable, clinical condition.

Treatment of acute chest pain begins with limitation of the factors that trigger angina, most notably exercise. Patients should be on **strict bedrest**, aided in some cases by gentle sedation. Further therapy aims to re-adjust the factors that determine oxygen supply and consumption. Intravenous infusions of **nitrate** are used in the relief of acute ischaemia and do so by a reduction in venous return (preload), a decrease in systemic blood pressure (afterload) and dilatation of coronary arteries.

β-Blockers and/or **calcium antagonists** are often used in the treatment of unstable angina. β-Blockers reduce oxygen demand by lowering heart

Pathology of unstable angina and myocardial infarction

In chronic stable angina pain is precipitated by exercise as narrowed coronary arteries are unable to increase their delivery of oxygen. The onset of symptoms in **unstable angina** and **myocardial infarction** is often sudden and unprovoked and it is thought that a similar event underlies the abrupt fall in coronary blood flow in these conditions. Alterations in the conformation of atherosclerotic plaques (such as ulceration or fissuring) are thought to be important in acute coronary artery occlusion. Endothelial and/or intimal damage provides a focus for platelet activation and subsequent formation of thrombus around the injured site. In unstable angina limited platelet aggregation and thrombosis occurs whereas in myocardial infarction a larger, more persistent thrombotic reaction develops.

It is likely that plaque damage is a necessary but not sufficient event for vascular occlusion and that additional factors influence the extent of the thrombotic reaction. Some people have more active thrombotic mechanisms and are said to be 'hypercoagulable'. For example smoking and high circulating catecholamine levels increase platelet reactivity. The presence of local and/or systemic thrombogenic risk factors at the time of plaque disruption may modify the extent and duration of thrombosis and account for the different pathological and clinical manifestations of acute coronary 'events'.

rate, reducing blood pressure and depressing myocardial contractility. Calcium antagonists reduce myocardial oxygen consumption by reducing systemic vascular resistance and coronary artery tone. The reflex tachycardia effect of nifedipine is usually prevented by the use of β-blockers. In patients where the use of β-blockers is prevented (such as people with heart failure or bronchospasm) the use of nifedipine should be avoided.

Intimal damage with superimposed thrombosis is usually the pathological cause of unstable angina. Such a stenosed artery is at risk of further, more serious occlusion if the thrombus extends. **Anticoagulation** with **intravenous heparin** is therefore mandatory in the management of unstable angina. **Aspirin** inhibits platelet activation at the site of intimal damage and should be given to all patients in whom there is no contraindication.

'Refractory' unstable angina

If, despite intensive pharmacological treatment, the symptoms of unstable angina persist then a state of refractory angina is said to exist. **Urgent angiography** is required to outline the coronary anatomy and locate the offending critical stenosis. If the lesion appears suitable for angioplasty or bypass grafting then one of these interventions is carried out urgently.

Treatment of unstable angina 'at a glance'

1. Relieve pain (opiates if necessary).
2. Aspirin.
3. Anticoagulate with heparin.
4. Intravenous nitrates.
5. β-Blockers and/or calcium antagonists.
6. If pain persists then consider referral to a cardiological centre for angiography.

MYOCARDIAL INFARCTION

This refers to the process in which an area of heart muscle dies because the artery supplying it has become occluded (Fig. 4.8). It usually occurs in patients with coronary artery atheroma when an already narrowed vessel is occluded by thrombus. There is often a history of angina, but in many patients myocardial infarction (MI) is the first presentation of coronary artery disease.

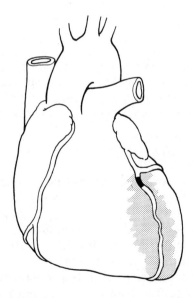

Fig. 4.8 Myocardial infarction. The area of muscle supplied by the occluded artery dies.

Clinical features

The cardinal feature of myocardial infarction is **pain**. This is similar to the pain of angina but is characteristically more severe, lasts longer and is not relieved by rest or sublingual nitrates. Reflex activation of the sympathetic autonomic nervous system often causes profuse sweating and patients frequently vomit. Pyrogens released by infarcted muscle may cause a low grade fever.

A significant minority of patients with myocardial infarction do not experience pain and in such cases the diagnosis is more difficult. The elderly, particularly, may have 'silent' infarcts; as may diabetics in whom autonomic neuropathy abolishes visceral pain sensation. These patients tend to present with one or more of the complications of myocardial infarction, such as heart failure or hypotension. In the elderly the only presenting feature may be confusion.

Physical signs in myocardial infarction relate to loss of a portion of functioning myocardium and the generalized activation of the autonomic nervous system that occurs as a reflex response to this. Patients look ill and grey and are generally **sweaty**, **clammy** and **tachycardic** as sympathetic activation causes peripheral vasoconstriction. Involvement of the pacemaking or conduction apparatus, however, may cause **bradycardia**. If a significant portion of the left ventricle is damaged then its output may be impaired. Right ventricular output rises along the Starling curve but the left ventricle cannot increase its rise in parallel. Pulmonary venous pressure rises and **acute pulmonary oedema** follows. Auscultation reveals **added heart sounds** and **basal lung crepitations**. A raised jugular venous pressure (JVP) may be seen in patients with significant right ventricular infarction.

Investigations

The history is of overwhelming importance in the diagnosis of myocardial infarction and usually provides sufficient information on which to base early management decisions. In addition there are two investigations that provide hard evidence for infarction.

Electrocardiographic (ECG) changes

In most cases of myocardial infarction a characteristic set of progressive ECG changes is produced which are the result of the abnormal electrical properties of dead/dying and ischaemic tissue (Fig. 4.9). The leads in which they occur indicate the area of damaged myocardium. Ventricular muscle depolarizes from endocardium to epicardium (from the inside out). An electrode placed in the cavity of a ventricle would register only a downward deflection (Q wave) since all ventricular impulses are moving away from the cavity. Infarcted myocardial tissue is electrically inert, so electrodes that 'look at' the area of infarcted myocardium behave as though they were placed

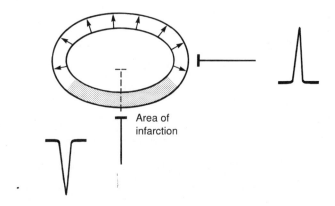

Fig. 4.9 Q waves. Infarcted tissue is electrically inert, so an electrode over an area of infarction behaves as if it were placed in the cavity. Myocardium depolarizes from endocardium to epicardium (inside out), so all impulses will be moving away from the cavity electrode. This produces a downward deflection (the Q wave). An electrode placed over an area of normal myocardium registers a positive deflection.

inside the cavity and record Q waves. In other words, dead tissue behaves as an electrical window through which electrodes may record intra-cavity potentials. Q waves that are ≥ 25% of the height of the ensuing R wave or ≥ one small square in breadth are considered to be pathological and suggest previous myocardial infarction (Fig. 4.10). Q waves in leads II, III and avF, for example, suggests previous inferior infarction (Fig. 4.11).

In the early stages of MI the infarcting muscle is still electrically active and there is no 'window' through which Q waves may be recorded. Ischaemic myocardium causes electrical abnormalities in the T waves and S–T segments of the ECG. The S–T segment corresponds to the onset and early part of ventricular repolarization and is usually isoelectric. Infarcting myocardium has abnormal repolarization properties which result in characteristic **elevation of the S–T segments** from the isolectric line and peaking of the **T waves** to form **arrowheads**. There may be depression of the S–T segments in the leads lying opposite to the area of infarction (reciprocal S–T depression). Following infarction the acute changes are replaced by **permanent Q waves** as described above. Abnormalities of the S–T segments usually return to normal within 3 days, but the **T waves often remain inverted permanently**.

Occasionally ECG changes are restricted to abnormalities of the S–T segment and T waves without the subsequent development of Q waves. This is termed '**non-Q wave**' or **subendocardial infarction** and it is thought that the area of infarction does not extend to the full thickness of the ventricular wall. The measurement of serial cardiac enzymes assumes a greater than normal role in the diagnosis of non-Q wave infarction and helps to distinguish it from unstable angina.

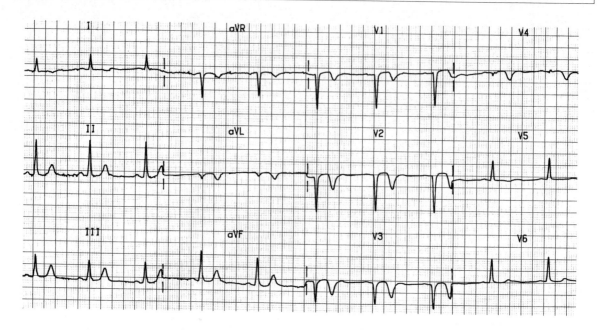

Fig. 4.10   ECG of a patient with previous anterior infarction. Note the Q waves in leads V_{2-4}.

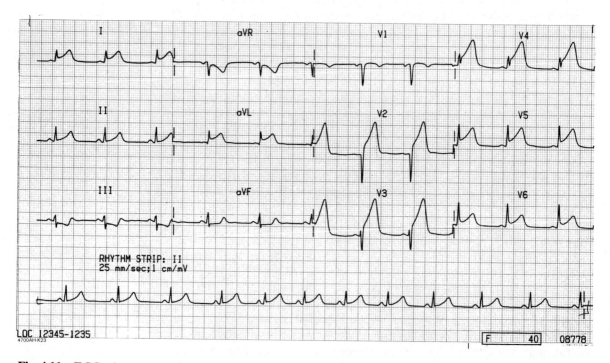

Fig. 4.11   ECG of a patient with acute antero-lateral infarction showing S–T elevation in leads I, aVL and V_{2-6}.

Cardiac enzymes

The rise in blood levels of the cellular enzymes released by dying myocardium may be used to help confirm the diagnosis of myocardial infarction. The three most commonly measured enzymes are **creatinine kinase (CK)**, **aspartate aminotransferase (AST)**, and **lactate dehydrogenase (LDH)**. The levels of these enzymes rise and fall at different and characteristic rates after infarction (Fig. 4.12). CK levels rise to exceed the normal range less than six hours after the onset of infarction, reach a peak within 24 hours and return to normal by 48 hours. It is the enzyme of most diagnostic use in the early stages of myocardial infarction but is of less value with increasing time after the onset of chest pain. CK is also produced by damaged skeletal muscle and brain so recent falls, intramuscular injections or convulsions may all produce false positive results. In recent years a number of different iso-enzymes have been identified. The myocardial version (**CK-MB**) is almost specific for damaged myocardium. AST levels peak between 24 and 48 hours and fall to normal after about 72. The number of false positives (AST is released by damaged erythrocytes, hepatocytes and kidneys) means its value is chiefly as part of a series of cardiac enzymes or for the purposes of confirming a diagnosis retrospectively. LDH peaks at 3–4 days and remains above the normal range for several days after that. Its use is similar to that of AST.

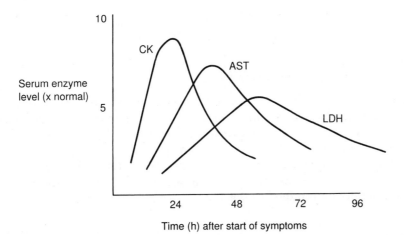

Fig. 4.12   The levels of cardiac enzymes with time following acute myocardial infarction.

Serum enzyme levels

Infarcting muscle releases intracellular enzymes into the blood that may be measured. The most useful of these, clinically, is **creatinine kinase (CK)** which is the first to become elevated. Raised enzyme levels are compatible with but not diagnostic of myocardial infarction. False positives (raised CK but no infarction) may be caused by injury to non-cardiac muscle such as occurs following falls or intramuscular injections.

Case history

An 80-year-old lady was found confused in her bed by her home help. She was brought to Casualty where she denied any symptoms. In particular she denied chest pain or shortness of breath. Physical examination was normal. A 12-lead ECG showed Q waves in leads II, II and aVF. Cardiac enzyme results were as follows:

	Day of admission	*Next day*
CK	435iu/l	120iu/l
AST	350iu/l	120iu/l

These results are typical of recent myocardial infarction. The CK is elevated but not dramatically so and this represents the downward part of the graph. The AST is 5 times the upper limit of normal and by the following day is less than half the original value. This lady has almost certainly had a silent myocardial infarction which is an important cause of confusion in the elderly. The presence of pathological Q waves in the inferior leads of the ECG suggests that inferior myocardial infarction was the cause of the confusion.

Treatment of myocardial infarction

Relief of symptoms, treatment to limit infarct size and prompt attention to complications such as arrhythmias and heart failure are the mainstays of the management of acute myocardial infarction. Patients must have **intravenous access** for the administration of emergency drugs and should be given **60% oxygen** as pO_2 falls during acute infarction. Pain is treated with opiates such as **diamorphine**. Nausea is treated with anti-emetics such as **metoclopramide** or **cyclizine**.

Thrombolysis

Thrombolysis is the breaking up and dissolution of blood clots and occurs naturally in the body. It may be augmented and accelerated by thrombolytic agents such as **streptokinase** and **tissue plasminogen activator (TPA)**. This is the basis of thrombolytic therapy in myocardial infarction which aims to recanalize the occluded coronary vessels, thereby minimizing myocardial damage. This theory is borne out in clinical practice. Many large multi-centre trials have shown reductions in mortality from myocardial infarction following thrombolysis.

Thrombolytic agents

Streptokinase is a bacterial product that activates the body's own fibrinolytic system by forming complexes with plasminogen (plasminogen forms plasmin which digests fibrin). These complexes activate more plasminogen molecules, eventually resulting in a state of hypofibrinogenaemia. **Tissue plasminogen activator (TPA)** is a naturally occurring substance that stimulates the conversion of plasminogen to plasmin. Many large, multi-centre trials have shown that thrombolytic therapy given to patients with acute myocardial infarction reduces early and late mortality. Results are better when thrombolysis is given within six hours of the onset of chest pain, but benefits may still be gained up to 12 hours after symptoms start. It is not clear which is the best thrombolytic for acute infarction. Some studies suggest that TPA may have a superior effect to SK, but it is more expensive and is usually reserved for young patients presenting early with anterior infarction.

Arrhythmias

The mortality from myocardial infarction is around 40%. Most of these deaths occur out of hospital and are largely the result of lethal arrhythmias such as ventricular fibrillation and ventricular tachycardia. Swift admission to hospital is crucial and patients should have **continuous ECG monitoring** on specialized coronary care units (**CCUs**), where nurses are trained to recognize arrhythmias and start resuscitation promptly. A defibrillator should always be available in the assessment area of the A&E department, during transfer of the patient and on the CCU.

Arrhythmias in myocardial infarction

Myocardial infarction may be complicated by any rhythm disturbance. The most important tachyarrhythmias are **ventricular tachycardia** and **ventricular fibrillation**. The latter requires immediate cardioversion with DC energy although occasionally a **praecordial thump** may restore sinus rhythm. Ventricular tachycardia associated with hypotension may also require DC shock, but if the patient is haemodynamically stable then intravenous **lignocaine** may be tried. Such ventricular arrhythmias occurring more than 24–48 hours after infarction are termed 'late' arrhythmias and carry a poor prognosis. Electrophysiological studies to guide therapy are usually required.

If the area of damage involves the pacemaking or conduction apparatus then **bradycardias** may result. Involvement of the AV node is usually due to **inferior infarction**. All degrees of AV block may be seen, but treatment with temporary pacing is required only if the patient is hypotensive. Conduction disturbances with inferior infarcts usually recover spontaneously, although this may take up to 10 days. The septum and bundle branches are supplied by the first branch of the left anterior descending artery, so conduction defects with **anterior infarction** suggest that occlusion of the LAD is very proximal and a large area of myocardium is in jeopardy. Heart block in this context usually requires temporary pacing and may even necessitate a permanent system later. Bundle branch block alone does not require pacing. The indications for temporary pacing in acute myocardial infarction are:

Inferior infarction	Heart block accompanied by hypotension
Anterior infarction	Complete heart block Mobitz type II Bifascicular block (RBBB usually with left axis deviation) Alternating right and left bundle branch block

Heart failure

Heart failure occurs in acute myocardial infarction because damage to a portion of myocardium reduces the amount of muscle available for contraction. In **anterior infarction** the anterior wall of the LV bears most of the damage, so that this chamber is unable to empty itself efficiently. The relatively normal RV continues to drive blood forward into the pulmonary circulation and fluid accumulates in the lungs resulting in **pulmonary oedema**. In **inferior infarction** the inferior (diaphragmatic) wall of the LV is often damaged but there may also be damage to the RV sufficient to impair its function. Poor RV emptying leads to high right-sided venous pressures. A raised JVP in the context of acute inferior infarction is not necessarily an indication for diuretics. In fact, by giving intravenous fluid (and thereby increasing right ventricular preload) it is sometimes possible to improve RV output along the Starling curve. However, this should be done cautiously as inferior myocardial infarction also damages the left ventricle and too much fluid may precipitate pulmonary oedema.

The anatomy of myocardial infarction

The heart is supplied by the right and left coronary arteries (Fig. 4.13). The **right coronary artery (RCA)** runs forward over the right atrium to descend in the atrioventricular (AV) groove. It usually gives rise to the **posterior descending artery** which runs in the posterior interventricular (IV) septum towards the apex. The **RCA** supplies mainly the right atrium (including the pacemaking apparatus), right ventricle and inferior left ventricular wall. **The left coronary artery (LCA)** arises from the posterior aspect of the aorta and passes behind pulmonary trunk. It divides into the **left anterior descending (LAD)** artery which runs in the IV groove down the front of the heart and **left circumflex artery** which occupies the posterior part of the AV groove. The LAD supplies mainly the anterior part of the LV wall and the left circumflex supplies the LA and lateral aspect of the LV.

With this in mind it is easy to see the basis of the typical ECG changes and complications associated with different areas of infarction. **RCA** occlusions lead to death of mainly **inferior (diaphragmatic) heart muscle** so the electrical changes are seen in those leads which examine this area (**II, III and aVF**). Damage to the pacemaking and AV conducting systems with inferior infarcts frequently causes **bradyarrhythmias** and **heart block**. Occlusions of the LAD may cause extensive loss of left ventricular muscle so antero-lateral myocardial infarction may be complicated by **acute left ventricular failure**. If the papillary muscles are damaged then prolapse of the mitral valve may occur, causing **acute mitral regurgitation** and **pulmonary oedema**. ECG changes in anterior infarction are found in the chest leads V_{1-4} and in lateral infarction in **I, aVL and V_{5-6}**.

Management of myocardial infarction 'at a glance'

1. Oxygen.
2. Intravenous cannula and administer opiate analgesia with anti-emetic.
3. Cardiac monitor.
4. 12-Lead ECG.
5. Aspirin 300 mg.
6. If thrombolysis indicated start without delay.
7. Send blood for cardiac enzymes, electrolytes, blood count.
8. CXR. Unless the suspicion of aortic dissection is high do not wait for CXR before starting thrombolysis.

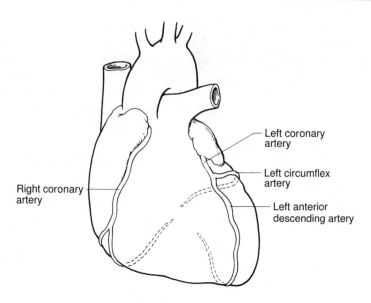

Fig. 4.13 The coronary circulation.

Other complications

Healing myocardium is weak and may rupture causing one of several effects. If the outer wall of the left ventricle ruptures then blood enters the pericardial sac (haemopericardium). The heart becomes 'squashed', diastolic filling is impaired and cardiac output falls acutely. This is called **cardiac tamponade** and most patients die suddenly.

Rupture of the interventricular septum establishes a communication between the two ventricles (**ventricular septal defect**). Rupture of the papillary muscles allows the mitral valve to 'balloon' back into the left atrium, causing torrential **mitral regurgitation**. Both of these conditions are characterized by acute heart failure with hypotension and a pansystolic murmur. It is difficult to distinguish the two clinically and **echocardiography** is required to make the diagnosis. Even with surgical intervention mortality is high.

If the area of myocardium damaged is very large then heart failure may exist in combination with hypotension and poor peripheral perfusion. This is called **cardiogenic shock**. It requires treatment with inotropes to support the heart and carries a poor prognosis. This condition is discussed in more detail in Chapter 3.

Myocardial damage may in turn cause inflammation of the pericardium. This may occur in the first few days after an infarct or develop several weeks later in association with fever and raised ESR (**Dressler's syndrome**). Non-steroidal anti-inflammatory drugs (NSAIDs) usually relieve symptoms in both cases, although in a few patients a short course of steroids may be needed.

Infarcted muscle heals by fibrosis. Scar tissue is weaker than healthy myocardium and if the healing process is not adequate then a localized bulge called a **ventricular aneurysm** may form at the site of the original infarct (Fig. 4.14). This may provide a focus for ventricular arrhythmias or be a site of clot formation with subsequent embolization. If either of these become problematical surgical excision of the aneurysm may be considered.

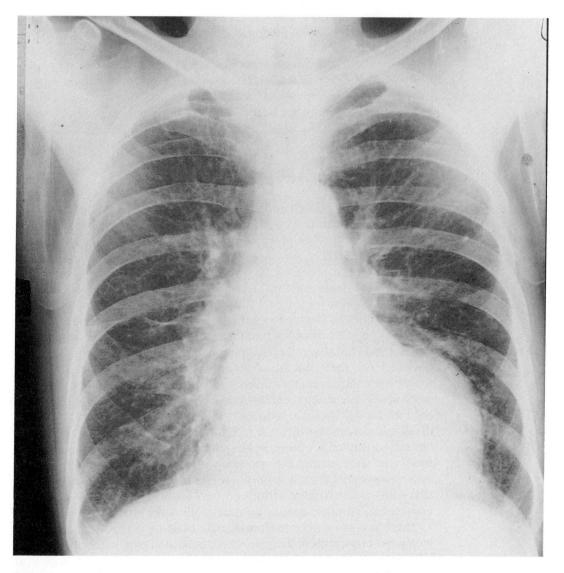

Fig. 4.14   Chest X-ray showing left ventricular aneurysm. Note the localized bulge of the left heart border. This patient also has left ventricular failure as a result of the aneurysm.

> **Case history**
> A 50-year-old man presented to Casualty with a 2-hour history of severe crushing central chest pain. On examination he was sweaty and unwell with a pulse of 100 beats/min and blood pressure 120/70 mmHg. A 12-lead ECG showed concave upwards S–T segment elevation in leads II, III and aVF.
>
> This man is having an acute inferior myocardial infarction. He should be given oxygen and attached to a cardiac monitor. Intravenous access should be established and he should be given opiate analgesia, an anti-emetic and aspirin. Having established that there are no contraindications to thrombolysis (recent surgery, active peptic ulceration, bleeding diathesis) he should be thrombolysed without delay. Unless there is any clinical suspicion of aortic dissection (interscapular pain or unequal pulses) there is no need to wait for a CXR before starting thrombolytic therapy. He requires continuous ECG monitoring on a Coronary Care Unit where arrhythmias can be monitored and treated promptly.

PREVENTATIVE CARDIOLOGY

The risk factors that predispose to coronary artery disease were discussed earlier in this chapter. Increasing emphasis is now placed on risk factor modification programmes both in General Practice and in the hospital setting.

Lipids

Opinion varies as to exactly what level of cholesterol justifies treatment, but most people advise six months of dietary modification for patients with a total cholesterol of >5.2 mmol/l. If diet alone does not have the desired effect then pharmacological treatment is added. The data from recent clinical trials suggest that a statin (such as simvastatin) is the agent of choice. These reduce endogenous cholesterol synthesis by inhibiting the enzyme HMG CoA reductase. In addition to lowering LDL these drugs cause a modest increase in HDL levels, which seems somehow to be 'cardioprotective'. Some angiographic studies have also shown that treatment with simvastatin reduces the number of new atheromatous lesions and may even cause partial regression of pre-existing ones. Fears that long-term treatment with cholesterol lowering therapy may increase non-coronary mortality have not been founded.

There is some evidence from clinical trials to suggest that long-term treatment of asymptomatic patients with isolated hypercholesterolaemia reduces morbidity or mortality from coronary artery disease. In clinical practice, however, the decision depends largely on the presence of other risk factors. Marked hyperlipidaemia in a young patient with a family history of early death from coronary artery disease, for example requires a more aggressive intervention than mild hypercholesterolaemia in an otherwise asymptomatic patient of 75.

Smoking

The evidence suggests that it is never too late to stop smoking. Patients may derive variable benefit from nicotine-flavoured chewing gum and support groups.

Hypertension

There is no firm 'cut-off' point for the treatment of hypertension. There is little evidence to suggest that pharmacological control of 'mild' hypertension in the absence of other risk factors has any effect on the incidence of coronary artery disease. However, with established disease and in the presence of other risk factors such as hypercholesterolaemia a more aggressive policy is justified.

Exercise

The value of exercise programmes, particularly following acute infarction, is controversial and has proved difficult to investigate scientifically. The data available suggest that exercise probably does have a beneficial effect in patients with impaired left ventricular function but it may be that the most important effect is on patient psychology with an overall feeling of 'well-being'. Most people agree that gentle, graded exercise has an important role to play in rehabilitation following myocardial infarction. Cardiac rehabilitation groups are important both in providing a stimulus to participate in exercise and in providing the opportunity for patients to see that they need not become limited by their condition.

5 Valvular heart disease

A schematic diagram of the pulmonary and systemic circulations is shown in Fig. 5.1. The co-ordinated actions of the valves in time with systole and diastole ensure that, in health, blood is directed from the right side of the heart through the lungs to the left heart and then into the aorta. Defects in valvular function cause one of two effects. If the aperture of a valve is narrowed (known as **stenosis**) then pressure in the chamber before the obstruction rises as a greater force is required to drive blood across the valve. This is known as **pressure loading** the heart. In contrast if a valve is leaky (**regurgitant** or **incompetent**) then blood leaking back into a chamber is added to the blood that arrives for the next cardiac cycle. The extra volume of blood causes that chamber to dilate. This is known as **volume loading** the heart.

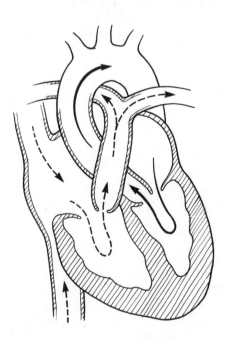

Fig. 5.1 Schematic diagram of the heart and pulmonary circulation, showing the four chambers, valves and direction of blood flow.

Abnormalities of valve function usually take several years to develop (exceptions to this include acute mitral regurgitation in myocardial infarction or infective endocarditis; and acute aortic regurgitation in aortic dissection or infective endocarditis). As the lesion progresses the heart 'adapts' to these abnormal pressures/volumes and the patient may remain asymptomatic. Such valvular lesions are said to be 'compensated'. For example in a patient with narrowing of the aortic valve (aortic stenosis) the left ventricle hypertrophies in order to be able to generate a greater head of pressure and drive blood across the stenosed valve into the aorta. Patients with aortic stenosis (AS) may remain well for years and require no medical attention. This chapter will focus mainly on disorders of the mitral and aortic valves as they are the commonest lesions. Tricuspid valve disease will be mentioned and is also discussed in Chapter 3.

MITRAL VALVE DISEASE

The mitral valve lies between the left atrium (LA) and the left ventricle (LV). So-called because of its resemblance to a Bishop's mitre it has two leaflets which are attached to a fibromuscular ring between the two chambers. Flow across the mitral valve in health occurs during diastole. Freshly oxygenated blood from the pulmonary veins flows more or less directly into the LV during the period of passive filling. This is followed by atrial contraction which provides an extra 'kick' to ventricular filling. During systole the mitral valve is held taut by the action of the chordae tendinae and the papillary muscles, thereby ensuring that blood is directed forward into the systemic circulation rather than back into the LA and pulmonary veins.

Mitral valve

Diastole: Open as blood flows into the ventricle from the lungs

Systole: Held shut by the chordae tendinae and papillary muscles

---

Mitral stenosis

This occurs almost exclusively as a result of previous **rheumatic fever**. There is progressive fusion of the two leaflets such that the aperture of the valve is narrowed and flow into the LV during diastole is reduced. The LA hypertrophies in order to force blood across the narrowed valve. Hence pressure in this chamber and in the pulmonary veins rises. It is important to realize that **left ventricular systolic function is normal**, but cardiac output is limited by the reduced flow of blood into the LV during diastole (Fig. 5.2).

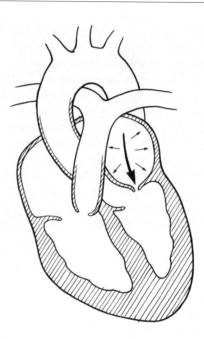

Fig. 5.2 Mitral stenosis.

Symptoms in mitral stenosis are attributable to two factors. Firstly, with exercise venous return to the right side of the heart increases and RV output rises (Starling's law). Pulmonary blood flow therefore rises, but flow into the LV across the mitral valve is limited. LA pressure tends to increase, leading to pulmonary venous congestion and **breathlessness**. Patients may also complain of **orthopnoea**. Secondly, the state of low cardiac output due to reduced LV filling may lead to **chronic fatigue**. It is not uncommon for mitral stenosis to present in pregnancy as a previously compensated lesion is exposed to increased circulatory demands. Sometimes the added burden of a chest infection is the precipitating factor. Another common precipitant is the onset of atrial fibrillation. As mitral stenosis progresses, LA size and pressure rise. Under such conditions atrial muscle may start to fibrillate. As the extra force of LA systole is lost LV filling (and therefore output) is further compromised. In addition if the ventricular response rate in AF is rapid, the heart spends proportionately less time in diastole and LV filling is reduced still further.

Examination in patients with MS reflects these haemodynamic changes. Patients may have the **chaotically irregular pulse** of atrial fibrillation. When the mitral valve closes it does so with increased force and may with time become palpable, felt as a **tapping apex beat**. Auscultation often reveals a **loud first sound** for the same reason. If the valve is still mobile (stenosed valves may calcify and become rigid with time) then it opens jerkily early in diastole due to the high LA pressures. This may be heard just after the second heart sound as a

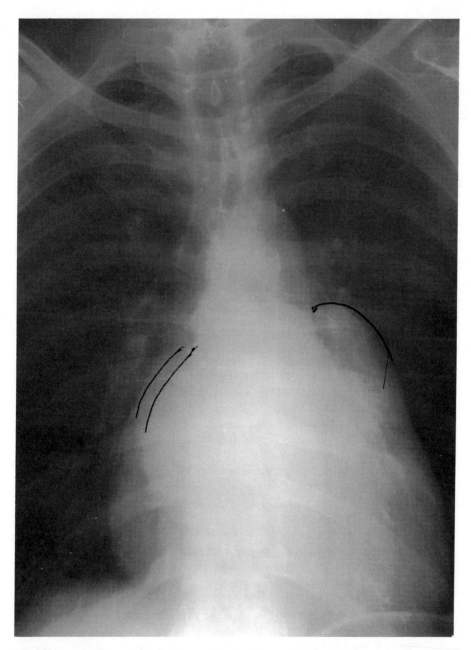

Fig. 5.3 Chest X-ray of a patient with mitral stenosis. Note the convex left heart border and the double shadow at the right heart border created by the enlarged left atrium.

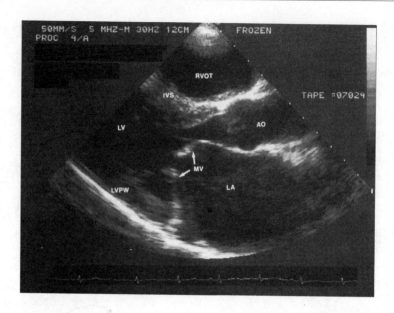

Fig. 5.4 Echocardiogram of a patient with mitral stenosis, showing thickened mitral valve leaflets (MV) with a narrowed aperture.

high-pitched **opening snap**. The **murmur** of mitral stenosis occurs in diastole and is a low-pitched, **rumbling** sound heard best at the apex. If the patient is in sinus rhythm there may be an increase in the intensity of the murmur just prior to the first heart sound as atrial contraction increases the turbulence across the valve. This is called **pre-systolic accentuation**.

Chest X-ray in mitral stenosis may show the double shadow of a large left atrium and evidence of pulmonary venous congestion (Fig. 5.3). Cardiomegaly, if present, is often due to RV dilatation consequent to pulmonary hypertension. There may be ECG evidence of LA hypertrophy, with a biphasic P wave in V_1 or a bifid P wave in the inferior leads. **Echocardiographic features** include thickened, rigid, fused mitral valve cusps with restricted movement (Fig. 5.4), LA enlargement and abnormal patterns of blood flow across the valve in diastole on Doppler studies.

Many patients with compensated mitral stenosis do not require treatment. If symptoms of exertional dyspnoea develop **medical** treatment includes **diuretics** to reduce fluid overload and **digoxin** to control the ventricular rate if the patient is in AF. Patients with AF due to mitral valve disease are particularly prone to thromboembolic complications such as stroke and require long term anticoagulation with **warfarin**. **Intervention** is reserved for those whose exercise tolerance is limited despite medical therapy. Options include dilating the valve orifice (either percutaneously with a balloon or surgically) and replacement with a prosthesis (for types of prostheses see page 107).

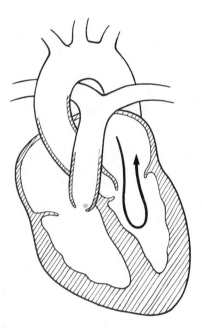

Fig. 5.5   Mitral regurgitation.

Mitral regurgitation

If the mitral valve is incompetent (regurgitant) then blood is misdirected back into the LA during systole, rather than forward into the aorta (Fig. 5.5). Consequently, in the diastole of the next cardiac cycle there is increased flow across the valve into the LV as the misdirected blood is added to normal pulmonary venous return. Since a proportion of stroke volume refluxes into the LA **total stroke volume** must increase if cardiac output is to be maintained. This **volume loads** the LV, which dilates and hypertrophies in order to accommodate the increased amount of blood. The LA dilates and AF is not uncommon.

   Symptoms are usually absent until LV failure supervenes. Raised left atrial and pulmonary venous pressures lead to **exertional dyspnoea** and **orthopnoea**. As with mitral stenosis the onset of atrial fibrillation may cause haemodynamic deterioration and, with time, lead to thromboembolic complications. If the mitral regurgitation is acute (see inset for causes of MR) then sudden haemodynamic deterioration occurs.

   Examination may reveal the **irregular pulse** of AF, the **displaced forceful apex beat** of a volume loaded LV and a **systolic murmur** heard at the apex and radiating into the axilla. This is usually **pansystolic**, but if the MR is due to a floppy mitral valve then the murmur may only be heard in late systole. Increased diastolic filling due to the regurgitant blood often produces a **third heart sound**.

Causes of mitral regurgitation

The mitral valve apparatus consists of the **annulus (ring)**, the **valve leaflets**, the **chordae tendinae** and the **papillary muscles**. The coordinate action of all these structures is required for the valve to be competent. Causes of mitral regurgitation can therefore be grouped according to which particular structure is malfunctioning.

Abnormalities of the leaflets	**Mitral valve prolapse** **Rheumatic heart disease** **Infective endocarditis**
Abnormalities of the ring	**Calcification of the mitral annulus** **Dilatation of the LV** (from any cause) may stretch the ring and render the valve incompetent
Papillary muscle/chordae tendinae dysfunction	If **myocardial infarction** involves the papillary muscles then the valve balloons back into the LA and MR results. Chordal rupture may complicate infective **endocarditis** and **Marfan's syndrome**

Mitral valve prolapse

This is a common condition, possibly affecting up to 5% of the population. The valve leaflets are excessively pliable and bulge back into the LA during systole, causing MR in some people. Most patients are asymptomatic but a few present with atypical chest pain or arrhythmias. The classical features on examination include a mid-systolic click and sometimes a late systolic murmur at the apex. Most patients require no treatment other than reassurance, but those patients with MR are at increased risk of endocarditis and should receive prophylactic antibiotics.

CXR in mitral regurgitation may show **cardiomegaly**, a **large LA** and a **calcified mitral valve**. **Echocardiography** with **Doppler studies** provides information about LA and LV size and function, identifies the regurgitant jet and may show vegetations in infective endocarditis. Where MR complicates myocardial infarction one or both leaflets may be seen to move dyscoordinately in systole due to papillary muscle rupture. Cardiac catheterization demonstrates regurgitation of dye into the LA, documents LV size and function and identifies co-existent coronary artery disease.

Medical treatment of mitral regurgitation includes **diuretics** to reduce pulmonary venous congestion. **ACE inhibitors** may improve symptoms in MR by reducing aortic pressure which favours flow of blood forward into the systemic circulation rather than back into the LA, as well as by

Case history

A 64-year-old man saw his GP because of tiredness and breathlessness when gardening. This had been troubling him for several months but had become more troublesome in the previous three weeks. During that time he had noticed his heart 'thumping' in his chest whenever he climbed stairs. He had also been having difficulty sleeping at night and was only able to get to sleep if he propped himself up with several pillows. Examination revealed atrial fibrillation with a rate of 120/minute, a displaced, forceful apex beat and a pansystolic murmur at the apex radiating into the axilla.

This man's symptoms are of left-sided heart failure and the most likely cause is mitral regurgitation. Although it is not possible to tell how long he has been in atrial fibrillation the deterioration in exercise tolerance and the palpitations during exercise suggest that the precipitant of symptoms is the onset of atrial fibrillation. He requires cardiological referral for investigation and assessment of his mitral valve, including routine blood tests, ECG, CXR and echocardiogram.

Treatment includes diuretics, digoxin to control the ventricular rate and anticoagulation with warfarin to reduce the risk of systemic emboli. ACE inhibitors may also be of benefit. If his symptoms cannot be controlled medically or there is evidence of left ventricular dysfunction on echo then he may require cardiac catheterization with a view to mitral valve replacement.

limiting activation of the renin–angiotensin system. If AF develops digoxin may be necessary. All patients with AF should be anticoagulated with warfarin unless contra-indicated.

Patients whose symptoms cannot be controlled medically or those who have worsening LV function require **mitral valve replacement or repair**. Acute mitral regurgitation (such as occurs with papillary muscle rupture in acute MI) requires urgent valve surgery.

AORTIC VALVE DISEASE

The aortic valve lies between the left ventricle and the root of the aorta and consists of three semilunar leaflets attached to a valve ring. It opens when systolic pressure in the LV exceeds that in the aorta and prevents the reflux of blood back into the LV during diastole when closed. Normal functioning of the aortic valve allows free flow of blood into the systemic circulation during systole and helps maintain blood pressure in diastole. Consequently, abnormalities of valve function may lead to important abnormalities of pulse pressure (the difference between systolic and diastolic values).

Aortic valve

Systole. Open as blood flows freely from LV into aorta

Diastole. Closed to prevent reflux of blood back into LV

Aortic stenosis (AS)

If the outlet of the LV is obstructed by a narrowed (stenosed) aortic valve then the LV must generate a greater pressure in order to open that valve (Fig. 5.6). This leads to **pressure loading** of the LV and a gradient is established across the aortic valve during systole. The ventricular wall undergoes compensatory **hypertrophy**, so that in the early stages cardiac output is maintained. However, with time and progressive narrowing of the valve aperture cardiac output falls off and symptoms of LV failure develop. Most cases of AS are caused by diffuse calcification either of a normal valve or one that is congenitally bicsuspid (with two leaflets). A few cases are due to previous rheumatic fever.

Causes of aortic stenosis

Calcification of the aortic valve (most cases)

Congenitally bicuspid valve (some cases)

Previous rheumatic fever (a few cases)

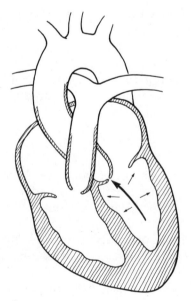

Fig. 5.6   Aortic stenosis.

Symptoms in AS are a function of reduced cardiac output and increased requirements of the hypertrophied LV for oxygen. With exercise RV output increases but the LV is unable to force blood across the stenosed valve. Consequently, LA and pulmonary venous pressures rise causing **exertional dyspnoea**. **Syncope** may be due either to arrhythmias or because cerebral perfusion becomes compromised by the inadequate cardiac output during exercise. Increased myocardial oxygen demand due to LV hypertrophy may cause **angina**. It must be stressed that symptoms occur late in the natural history of aortic stenosis. If intervention is delayed for too long then irreversible left ventricular failure or sudden death may occur.

Signs in AS include a carotid pulse which has a prolonged, slow upstroke (often called a **slow rising pulse**) as more time is required for the LV to eject its load. The hypertrophied ventricle may be felt as a **forceful apex beat** and the turbulent flow across the aortic valve may produce a **praecordial systolic thrill**. The gradient across the valve is maximal midway through systole, so that the **murmur** of AS starts quietly, crescendoes and then dies away again. It usually has a harsh quality and radiates into the carotids. If the valve is heavily calcified then the aortic component of the second heart sound will be quiet or even inaudible.

Important **investigations** in AS include an **ECG** which shows features of LV hypertrophy and a **CXR** which may show a calcified valve and dilatation of the aorta distal to the obstruction. **Echocardiography** usually shows a thickened, non-mobile aortic valve (Fig. 5.7), a hypertrophied LV and Doppler studies help estimate the gradient

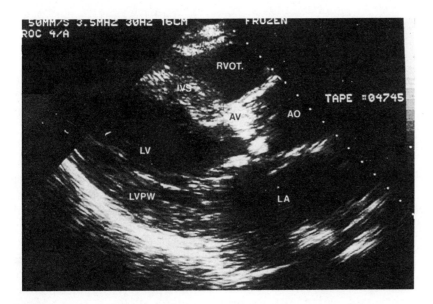

Fig. 5.7 Echocardiogram of a patient with aortic stenosis. Note the thickened, calcified aortic valve.

Case history

A 64-year-old lady collapsed unconscious while choosing some clothes in a department store. By the time the shop assistant arrived she had recovered a little and was able to sit in a chair with help. She insisted that her 'faint' was due to the hot weather and lack of air-conditioning in the shop but was persuaded to attend hospital where a Casualty doctor noted a small volume carotid pulse and an ejection systolic murmur that radiated into the neck. A 12-lead ECG showed left ventricular hypertrophy.

It is imperative to exclude aortic stenosis in this lady. Syncope in patients with aortic stenosis is a sinister symptom and may be the forerunner of sudden death. She requires urgent echocardiography and may need cardiac catheterization to document the pressure gradient across the aortic valve and examine the coronary arteries prior to aortic valve replacement. In a young patient with a low probability of coronary disease cardiac catheterization is often unnecessary if the Doppler study confirms significant AS.

The pressures documented at cardiac catheterization were as follows:

Pressure	(mmHg)
RA	4
RV	30/0
PA	32/18
PA (wedge)	12
LV	180/8
Aorta	100/70

These are typical pressure readings of aortic stenosis. There is a gradient of 80 mmHg across the aortic valve (normally there should be no gradient as blood flows freely across the valve). This lady's symptoms improved following aortic valve replacement.

across the valve from the velocity of blood flow. Cardiac catheterization is necessary where diagnostic uncertainty exists following echocardiography or if co-existent coronary artery disease is suspected. Pressure readings in the LV and proximal aorta allow the gradient across the valve to be measured (Fig. 5.8).

Treatment of AS is surgical with valve replacement and is undertaken if the patient has symptoms such as exertional dyspnoea, angina or syncope. Many cardiologists also recommend valve replacement in asymptomatic patients with a peak systolic gradient of 60 mmHg or more.

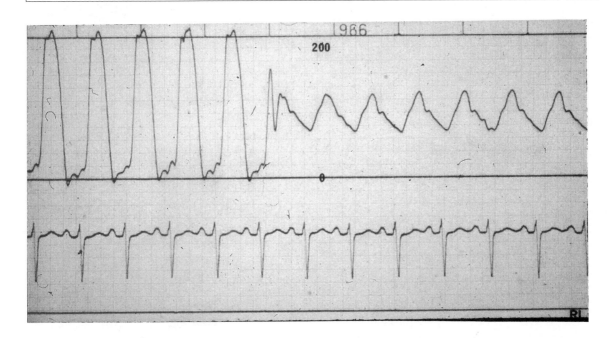

Fig. 5.8 LV and aortic pressure tracings of a patient with aortic stenosis. Note that the peak LV systolic pressure is much greater than peak aortic systolic pressure, indicating a pressure gradient across the aortic valve.

Aortic regurgitation

In this condition blood flows back across a 'leaky' aortic valve into the left ventricle during diastole (Fig. 5.9). This overloads the LV, which compensates by increasing its force of contraction and stroke volume. In the early stages of aortic regurgitation (AR) the LV copes well with this added burden but with time its function may become impaired and LV failure may supervene. This is not inevitable and the outcome depends on the severity of the regurgitation.

Symptoms in AR depend on the speed of onset of the lesion. If aortic regurgitation occurs acutely then there is no time for the LV to undergo the compensatory mechanisms of hypertrophy and dilatation and **acute LV failure** with **pulmonary oedema** occurs. Patients with chronic AR are usually asymptomatic until the LV begins to fail, when **exertional dyspnoea**, **fatigue** and **orthopnoea** develop. The increased oxygen demands of the overloaded LV may cause **angina**.

Examination in AR may reveal strikingly vigorous pulsations of the carotid arteries in the neck due to the large stroke volume (Corrigan's sign). The incompetent aortic valve is unable to maintain diastolic blood pressure and the effect is a pulse that seems to slap against the fingers if they are wrapped around the wrist with the patient's arm in the air. This is often called a 'collapsing pulse'. Regurgitation of blood into the LV

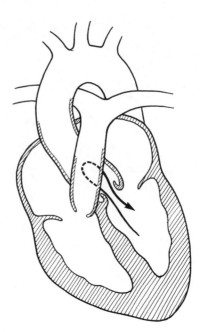

Fig. 5.9 Aortic regurgitation.

during diastole leads to enlargement of the ventricle which may be felt as a **displaced apex beat** with a prominent impulse. Blood flow back across the aortic valve is maximal early in diastole when pressure in the aortic root is at its highest and declines as blood runs off into the systemic circulation and aortic pressure falls. Consequently the **murmur** of AR is loudest early in diastole and then decrescendoes. It is best heard at the left sternal edge with the patient sitting forward in full expiration.

Incompetence of the aortic valve may be due to disease of the valve leaflets or secondary to dilatation of the aortic root. Leaflet disorders include **rheumatic disease**, **infective endocarditis** (either past or current) and **congenital** abnormalities such as a **bicuspid valve** (normal aortic valves have three cusps). **Calcified valves** may become regurgitant as well as stenotic. Diseases that cause dilatation of the aortic root and valve ring include **hypertension**, **Marfan's syndrome**, **aortic dissection** (Chapter 11) and certain connective tissue disorders such as **ankylosing spondylitis**.

There may be evidence of left ventricular hypertrophy on **ECG** and dilatation of the aortic root on **CXR**. **Echocardiography** can measure the diameter of the aortic root and Doppler studies identify the abnormal regurgitant jet. Patients being considered for valve replacement usually require **cardiac catheterization** to assess the severity of AR and outline the anatomy of the coronary arteries and aortic root.

AR is tolerated well until left ventricular dysfunction supervenes. **Diuretics** may improve symptoms of dyspnoea and **ACE inhibitors** may prevent ventricular dilatation and delay the need for surgical intervention. The onset of symptoms in AR is usually the indication for **valve replacement**, before there is irreversible left ventricular dysfunction. All patients with aortic regurgitation require antibiotic prophylaxis.

Tricuspid regurgitation

The tricuspid valve lies between the RA and RV and, as its name suggests, has three leaflets. Blood flows across the valve in diastole and, if the valve is competent, is prevented from refluxing into the RA during systole. Most cases of TR are due to a **stretched valve ring** due to chronic right heart failure and RV dilatation (often termed '**functional regurgitation**'), often secondary to pulmonary hypertension, but **rheumatic heart disease** and **endocarditis** are other causes. Reflux of blood into the RA leads to increased diastolic filling with the next cardiac cycle as the misdirected blood is added to systemic venous return during the next cardiac cycle (Fig. 5.10). Consequently, the RV becomes **volume overloaded** and dilated in a manner similar to LV dilatation in MR.

   Signs are therefore mainly of right heart failure, with **raised venous pressures** and **ankle oedema**. The regurgitant jet leads to striking systolic pulsations in the JVP called **'v' waves**. The **liver** is usually **enlarged** and is often **pulsatile** due to reflux of blood back into the RA, inferior vena cava and hepatic veins. If the TR is functional then there may be

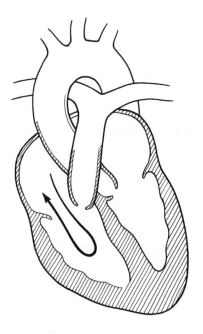

Fig. 5.10   Tricuspid regurgitation.

evidence of **pulmonary hypertension**, with a **right ventricular heave** and an accentuated P_2.

Investigations that help in the diagnosis of TR include an **ECG**, which may show evidence of RV hypertrophy and strain, a **CXR** which may show large pulmonary arteries from pulmonary hypertension and **echocardiography** which identifies the regurgitant jet. Doppler studies can estimate the pulmonary artery pressures. If these are elevated a diagnosis of functional TR can be made.

Treatment of TR is almost always medical with **diuretics** to reduce RV volume. TV replacement is occasionally required.

Tricuspid stenosis

This is very rare and generally occurs in combination with mitral stenosis secondary to previous rheumatic disease. A pressure gradient is established across the tricuspid valve akin to the gradient across the mitral valve in MS, causing symptoms and signs of right heart failure. The RA contracts vigorously in order to force blood across the stenotic valve, causing prominent 'a' waves in the jugular venous pulse. Treatment is usually with diuretics, but occasionally surgical valvotomy or replacement is required.

Pulmonary valve disease

The pulmonary valve lies between the RV and the pulmonary trunk. Diseases of the pulmonary valve are comparatively rare. **Pulmonary stenosis** is almost always congenital and is usually discovered because of an ejection systolic murmur heard in the pulmonary area on routine examination. It is discussed more fully in Chapter 10. In **pulmonary regurgitation** blood ejected into the pulmonary circulation refluxes back into the RV during diastole. It most commonly occurs as a result of pulmonary hypertension and is usually well tolerated.

SURGICAL OPTIONS IN THE TREATMENT OF VALVULAR LESIONS

When medical management of a valvular lesion fails, surgical intervention may be considered. Various options exist and the choice often depends on the degree of valvular dysfunction and the presence of complicating factors such as calcification and secondary pulmonary hypertension. Timing of surgery is difficult. The aim is to replace the diseased valve and restore normal haemodynamics before LV dysfunction or secondary pulmonary hypertension develop. However all types of valve replacement carry certain disadvantages as discussed below.

Valvotomy is the term given to surgical separation of the valve leaflets where they are causing stenosis and is most commonly used in mitral stenosis. Valvotomy may be either open or closed, but both require thoracotomy under general anaesthesia. In closed valvotomy a dilator is introduced through an incision in the LA and passed across the mitral valve. This procedure does not require cardio-pulmonary bypass and is suitable for patients with mobile, non-calcified, non-regurgitant valves. **Open valvotomy** involves surgical dissection of the leaflets under direct vision and is done under formal cardiopulmonary bypass.

Dilatation of native mitral valves has now largely been replaced by **balloon valvuloplasty**. A balloon is introduced percutaneously and passed across the stenosed valve in the deflated state. The leaflets are then divided by inflation of the balloon. This procedure avoids the need for cardiac surgery and, like valvotomy, is best reserved for non-calcific, non-regurgitant stenosed mitral valves. Stenosed aortic valves are nearly always calcified and do not dilate satisfactorily.

Often diseased valves are not suitable for balloon dilatation or valvotomy and a replacement valve is required. There are two main types: biological (tissue) valves obtained from other animal species and valves manufactured from metals or plastics. Tissue grafts do not require anti-coagulation but usually degenerate after 10 years, when a second (higher risk) replacement operation is then required. Artificial prostheses last longer but are thrombogenic and lifelong anticoagulation is required with the attendant risk of gastrointestinal and intracranial haemorrhage. Occasionally valves, especially a regurgitant mitral valve, can be repaired.

RHEUMATIC FEVER AND RHEUMATIC HEART DISEASE

Acute rheumatic fever is an inflammatory condition that affects a small percentage of young people with group A streptococcal pharyngitis. Antibodies to the streptococcus appear to cross-react with various tissues including the heart, skin, joints and brain causing an acute 'connective tissue type' illness, 2–3 weeks after infection. Clinical features include fever, arthralgia/arthritis, subcutaneous nodules rather like those seen in rheumatoid arthritis, a characteristic rash called erythema marginatum and bizarre involuntary restless movements known as chorea. Cardiac involvement is usually present in the acute stages and includes pericarditis, myocarditis, ECG changes such as first degree heart block and valvular lesions manifested as new or changed murmurs.

The incidence of rheumatic fever has declined dramatically in recent years, largely due to the wide availability of effective antibiotic therapy for paediatric pharyngitis. Where untreated streptococcal infections progress to established rheumatic fever, **treatment** centres around **bedrest**, **aspirin** for fever and arthralgia and **penicillin** to eradicate streptococcus. **Prophylactic penicillin** is required to the age of 25 or for a minimum of 5 years if the patient is 20 or more at the time of diagnosis.

Duckett Jones criteria for the diagnosis of acute rheumatic fever

The diagnosis of acute rheumatic fever is a notoriously difficult one, partly as it is becoming so uncommon and partly as the symptoms and their severity are so variable. In an attempt to standardize the diagnostic criteria Duckett Jones, an American physician, drew up a list of manifestations of acute rheumatic illness. In a patient with evidence of recent streptococcal infection (e.g. positive throat swabs or elevated ASO titre) the presence of two major or one major plus two minor criteria suggest a high likelihood of acute rheumatic fever in that patient.

Major criteria	Minor criteria
Carditis (new murmurs, pericardial effusion)	Fever
	Arthralgia
Polyarthritis	Raised ESR or CRP
Erythema marginatum	Previous rheumatic fever
Chorea	First degree heart block
Subcutaneous nodules	

Of those patients that have had an episode of acute rheumatic fever, over 50% will go on to develop chronic valvular disease. Chronic rheumatic valve disease most commonly affects the mitral and aortic valves, with variable stenosis and incompetence. Healing following acute valvulitis leads to scarring with or without calcification, and the various clinical manifestations as described earlier in this chapter.

INFECTIVE ENDOCARDITIS

As its name implies this condition is characterized by inflammation of the lining of the heart secondary to infection. In practice this rarely involves the lining of the heart chambers and this section will deal only with infections of the valvular structures. Most cases of infective endocarditis occur in patients with pre-existing valvular/congenital heart disease or in those with valve prostheses. However, groups of patients at risk of developing endocarditis in a previously normal heart include the elderly, intravenous drug abusers and the immunocompromised.

Clinical features are due in part to the central cardiac process and its haemodynamic consequences, but also to the systemic effects of the primary inflammatory process.

Systemic features include fever, sweats, arthralgia and malaise. Immune complex formation and deposition may produce splinter haemorrhages, **splenomegaly** and a focal **glomerulonephritis** with microscopic **haematuria**. Embolization of vegetations may occur,

Pathology of infective endocarditis

Organisms gain access to the heart valves via the bloodstream but only a minority of patients with bacteraemia go on to develop endocarditis. Common portals of entry include **dental surgery** (streptococcus viridans), **peripheral veins** (staphylococci) and the **genitourinary tract** (streptococcus faecalis). Bacteria (most commonly) or fungi seed the edges of heart valves, leading to an inflammatory reaction, platelet accumulation, fibrin deposition and the formation of a mass of avascular tissue known as a **vegetation**. The infecting organism effectively becomes sealed off from the host's immune mechanisms and from antibiotics, thereby allowing the destructive process to 'grumble on'. In the case of *Staphylococcus aureus* endocarditis this process is usually aggressive, leading rapidly to valve destruction and heart failure. Streptococcal, staphylococcal epidermidis and fungal endocarditis tend to cause a lower grade, insidious illness.

causing pulmonary embolism (from right-sided lesions) and metastatic abscesses in the brain or elsewhere (left-sided lesions). Local abscess formation is a particular feature of aortic valve vegetations, leading to **heart block** by damaging the conducting system in the interventricular septum.

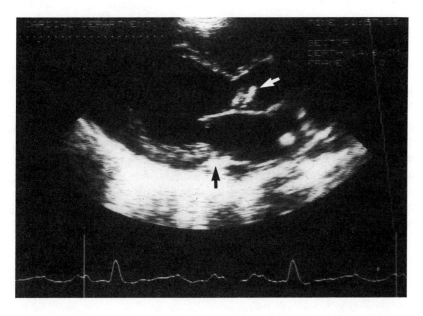

Fig. 5.11 Echocardiogram of a patient with infective endocarditis showing vegetations (arrowed) on the mitral and aortic valves. There is also a clot in the left atrium.

Cardiac features include the insidious onset of left- or right-sided heart failure, depending on the site of the infection and the development of new heart murmurs, usually regurgitant (aortic, mitral or tricuspid).

Helpful laboratory findings in endocarditis include normocytic normochromic anaemia, high white cell count, raised ESR and positive blood cultures. **Transthoracic and transoesophageal echocardiography** helps confirm valvular dysfunction and identifies vegetations, but if they are not seen the diagnosis is not excluded (Fig. 5.11).

The causative agent in infective endocarditis is partly shielded from antibiotic therapy by the avascular mass of tissue that makes up the vegetation. Consequently the treatment of endocarditis involves 'bathing' the infected valves in high doses of antibiotics for several weeks. Most cases of endocarditis are due to streptococcus, so it is sensible to start treatment with benzylpenicillin and low-dose gentamicin which are synergistic in their action against streptococcus. Further choice of antibiotic is guided by the results of blood cultures. Where staphylococcus is strongly suspected (e.g. in drug abusers or following valve replacement) treatment should include flucloxacillin and fucidic acid. Treatment is generally continued for a minimum of four weeks in uncomplicated cases and for six weeks for infected prosthetic valves.

Surgery may be required if there is evidence of progressive valve destruction with worsening heart failure; abscess formation; or large vegetations as these may embolize. It is preferable to eradicate the infection prior to operation but the timing of surgery depends on the clinical circumstances.

Antibiotic prophylaxis

For patients with congenital/valvular heart disease or prosthetic valves it is necessary to provide protection with antibiotics at the time of bacteraemia during non-sterile procedures such as dental extraction, cystoscopy or endoscopy. Current practice is that patients undergoing dental work receive 3 g of oral amoxycillin one hour prior to the procedure. Erythromycin is an alternative in those sensitive to penicillin. Patients undergoing cystoscopy or colonoscopy require antibiotic prophylaxis only if they have a prosthetic valve or have had a previous episode of endocarditis. Amoxycillin and intramuscular gentamicin is most often used, with vancomycin as an alternative in patients allergic to penicillin.

Arrhythmias 6

Disturbances of the heart's normal sinus rhythm are called **arrhythmias**. The heart may beat quickly, called a **tachycardia**, or slowly, when it is known as a **bradycardia**. In addition, sinus rhythm may be interrupted by extra heart beats, known as **extra-systoles** or **ectopic beats**.

TACHYCARDIAS

Tachycardias are generally accepted as being greater than 100 beats/minute. They may originate from anywhere in the heart, but are conventionally grouped into those arising from the ventricles (called **ventricular tachycardias**) and those that originate in structures lying above the ventricle (sinus node, atria or AV node) called **supraventricular tachycardias** (SVT). Some tachycardias arise out of abnormal connections between the atria and the ventricles. These are called **atrio-ventricular re-entrant tachycardias**, but are considered as part of the supraventricular tachycardia group.

Supraventricular tachycardias

Sinus tachycardia

The sinus node is the dominant natural pacemaker of the heart. Its normal rate of depolarization is 60–100 beats/minute and this is largely under autonomic control. Vagal stimulation causes slowing of the heart rate, whereas vagal inhibition or sympathetic stimulation cause the rate to increase. Thus, the development of a sinus tachycardia is a normal response to exercise, excitement, pain, shock or hypovolaemia, when sympathetic activation is high. It is unusual to see a sinus tachycardia greater than 180 beats/minute. Electrocardiographically it is recognized by the presence of a P wave before each QRS complex. The P waves have a similar morphology (shape) as during slower sinus rhythm because the site of impulse generation and the subsequent direction of spread is normal (Fig. 6.1). When sinus tachycardia occurs in the context of illness treatment is aimed at the underlying cause.

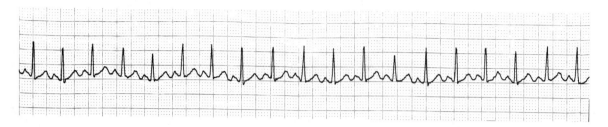

Fig. 6.1 Sinus tachycardia. Normal P waves and QRS complexes at a rate of 130/min.

Atrial fibrillation

Atrial fibrillation (AF) is the commonest pathological rhythm disturbance encountered and is a particularly common problem in the elderly.

Atrial fibrillation

AF is due to multiple areas of spontaneous electrical activity within the atria. Hundreds of small waves of depolarization begin to spread throughout the atria but end blindly when they encounter adjacent muscle fibres that have already been activated and are therefore **refractory**. This produces three important effects on the heart and circulation. First, the atria shimmer like a 'bag of worms' and do not produce the usual late diastolic 'mechanical kick' to ventricular filling. In some patients with poor ventricular function this can cause a reduction in cardiac output sufficient to aggravate or precipitate cardiac failure. Second, the atrio-ventricular node is bombarded by 300–600 impulses per minute and this may produce too rapid a ventricular response. Third, atrial fibrillation is associated with an **increased risk of stroke**. The lack of mechanical atrial systole predisposes to the formation of clots within the atria, which may embolize into the systemic circulation.

AF has many causes and almost any structural cardiac disorder may produce this rhythm. Common causes include **ischaemic heart disease, hypertension, rheumatic heart disease, post-cardiac surgery, cardiomyopathy** and **chronic lung disease. Thyrotoxicosis** is an important but relatively uncommon cause of AF. **Excess alcohol** often causes AF and, although this may be associated with a dilated type of cardiomyopathy (see Chapter 8), many patients with alcohol-induced AF have otherwise normal cardiac function. Many patients have no obvious underlying cause and are said to have **idiopathic** or **'lone' AF**. This diagnosis is made by excluding all other causes.

Atrial fibrillation may be asymptomatic and only diagnosed after the pulse has been taken for some other reason. The pulse has a chaotic

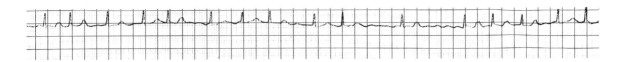

Fig. 6.2 Atrial fibrillation. Note the undulating baseline (fibrillary waves) and the irregularly spaced QRS complexes.

rhythm and there is often a discrepancy between the rate counted at the wrist and that auscultated at the apex. This is because stroke volume is partly determined by diastolic filling time. If there has been inadequate ventricular filling during diastole then the subsequent stroke volume will be small. Thus, some LV contractions will not eject sufficient blood to produce a palpable radial pulse. An ECG confirms the diagnosis, showing absent P waves and an isoelectric line disturbed by undulating fibrillary or 'f' waves. The QRS complexes are, like the pulse, irregularly spaced (Fig. 6.2).

Many patients are symptomatic and this is often determined by the rate of ventricular response. Patients may complain of palpitations and some can describe their irregularity. If there is underlying left ventricular dysfunction AF may precipitate or aggravate congestive cardiac failure for the reasons described above. In patients with underlying coronary artery disease AF may present with **angina**. A rapid ventricular response rate means that the heart has to do more 'work' and requires more oxygen. If there is coronary artery disease then myocardial blood supply may be insufficient to meet this increased oxygen demand. In addition, coronary blood flow occurs mainly during diastole, when the coronary arteries are no longer compressed by the contracting myocardium. At faster heart rates the heart spends less time in diastole so coronary blood flow is reduced.

The management of atrial fibrillation involves, where possible, treatment of the underlying cause such as abstention from alcohol or correction of thyrotoxicosis. **Echocardiography** may identify poor left ventricular function or mitral valve disease, but will also measure the size of the left atrium. The chances of a permanent return to sinus rhythm are much less if there is underlying structural cardiac disease, if the left atrium is grossly enlarged, or if atrial fibrillation has been present for a long time. If, for one of these reasons, it is thought unlikely that the patient will remain in sinus rhythm then therapy is aimed at controlling the ventricular response rate with drugs that block conduction through the AV node such as **digoxin**, **verapamil**, **diltiazem** or β-**blockers**. Warfarin (preferably) or aspirin are used to minimize the risk of stroke.

In many patients, however, consideration should be given to restoring sinus rhythm. If the ventricular rate is so rapid that the patient is hypotensive then **DC cardioversion** should be performed immediately. Most patients are not so unwell and in such cases early cardioversion may be attempted if the AF is of very recent onset (<48 hours). Cardioversion may be **electrical** (with DC energy) or **chemical** (with intravenous flecainide or amiodarone). Digoxin is ineffective in restoring sinus rhythm. There is a risk of thromboembolic problems following cardioversion, particularly if AF has been present for more than a few days, so most authorities recommend anticoagulation with warfarin for a period of 3–4 weeks prior to and after cardioversion so as to discourage atrial clot formation.

Once sinus rhythm has been restored, prophylactic therapy may be given to minimize the risk of developing further episodes of AF. In general, no treatment is given for a single attack, but if the patient has repeated episodes then prophylaxis with drugs that 'stabilize' the atrium may be tried. Commonly used drugs include **flecainide**, **sotalol** and **amiodarone**, although each has its drawbacks. Sotalol has a β-blocking action and is unsuitable for patients with bronchospasm or severe left ventricular dysfunction. Flecainide is also negatively inotropic and has been implicated in increased mortality in patients with ischaemic heart disease. Digoxin, verapamil and diltiazem are of little benefit in preventing atrial fibrillation. Amiodarone should be reserved for resistant cases because of its side-effect profile of **thyroid**, **liver** and **lung dysfunction** and **skin photosensitivity**. Occasionally if the ventricular rate cannot be controlled with medication or if drug therapy is not tolerated, then the AV node may be destroyed using a technique called **catheter ablation** (this technique is described later). This does not prevent atrial fibrillation, but by creating complete AV block it prevents the rapid and irregular heart rhythm that some patients find so distressing. An adequate ventricular rate is provided by implanting a pacemaker.

Case history

A 21-year-old male medical student presents to Casualty with sudden onset of fast, irregular palpitations. He had recently finished his pre-clinical examinations and for the previous week had been drinking heavily, consuming up to seven pints of beer a night. Examination revealed a chaotic pulse of 160 beats/min., but was otherwise unremarkable. An ECG showed atrial fibrillation with a mean ventricular response rate of 160/min.

Acute atrial fibrillation is a not uncommon consequence of excessive alcohol intake and is the likeliest cause in this patient. When AF is of very recent onset it is safe to cardiovert without prior anticoagulation with warfarin as the risk of thromboembolism is low. Following cardioversion thyroid function should be checked and he should have an echocardiogram to check that the heart is structurally normal. He should be informed that alcohol was the cause of the onset of AF and be warned about the dangers of continued excessive intake.

Atrial flutter

Although less common than atrial fibrillation, this arrhythmia is encountered in similar circumstances and with a similar presentation.

Atrial flutter

In this rhythm disorder there is a re-entrant circuit low down in the right atrium which leads to atrial activation at a rate of 300/min. In contrast to AF **the atria contract coordinately** which creates P waves but, because atrial depolarization does not originate in the sinus node, they do not have the same shape as during sinus rhythm. Each abnormally shaped P wave is called a **flutter wave** and at a rate of 300/min. the effect is to create a **'sawtooth'** pattern on the ECG, as shown in Fig. 6.3. Each 'tooth' represents an atrial contraction. The AV node is bombarded with 300 impulses/min. but is rarely able to conduct at such a fast rate and a degree of **AV block** exists. Most commonly the AV node conducts every other atrial impulse (**2 : 1 block**), leading to a ventricular rate of 150/min. For this reason atrial flutter should always be suspected in any patient with a regular, narrow complex tachycardia at this rate. If the atria conducts every third impulse 3 : 1 block exists; if every fourth then 4 : 1 and so on. The 'sawtooth' flutter waves are often best seen in the inferior leads (II, III and aVF) but frequently some of the flutter waves are hidden in the QRS complexes. If the diagnosis is in doubt careful **carotid sinus massage** or intravenous **adenosine** may be used. This transiently increases the degree of AV node blockade, the QRS complexes separate further on the ECG and the flutter waves become obvious.

Management follows similar principles to atrial fibrillation. Every effort should be made to restore sinus rhythm if possible. This nearly always requires **DC cardioversion** as pharmacological methods are usually unsuccessful. Once sinus rhythm is restored drugs such as **sotalol**, **flecainide** and **amiodarone** may be used to prevent recurrences. If these are ineffective then chronic atrial flutter is accepted and treatment is aimed at controlling the ventricular rate with AV nodal blocking drugs such as **digoxin**, **verapamil** or **β-blockers**.

Atrio-ventricular nodal re-entrant tachycardia

Atrio-ventricular nodal re-entrant tachycardia (AVNRT) is a common cause of paroxysmal (episodic and usually unpredictable supraventricular tachycardia in patients of all ages (Fig. 6.4). It is a benign condition although recurrent attacks can be troublesome.

Patients usually present with palpitations and can often describe the sudden onset and offset as well as their regularity. Occasional patients

(a)

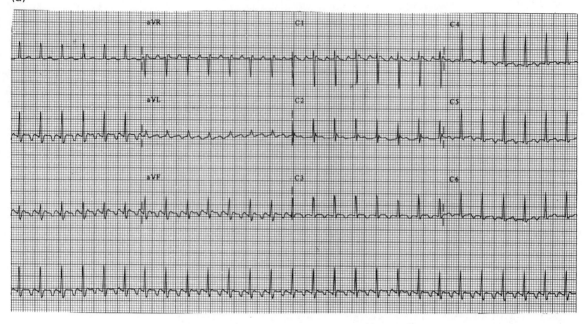

(b)

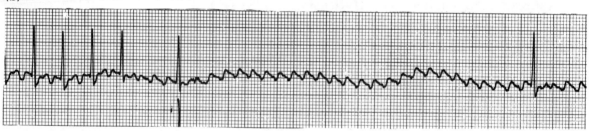

Fig. 6.3 Atrial flutter. Note the sawtooth appearance of the baseline with a flutter frequency of 300/min. (a) The QRS complexes have a rate of 150/min., so alternate flutter waves are conducted. Following intravenous adenosine (b) there is transient AV nodal block and the flutter waves become more obvious.

may be unaware of their rapid heart rate but feel breathless or even complain of chest discomfort (this does not necessarily indicate ischaemic heart disease as many such patients have normal coronary arteries). Contrary to popular belief polyuria (due to release of atrial natriuretic peptide during tachycardia) is uncommon. Precipitating factors include stress, tiredness, excess caffeine, alcohol ingestion and, in some women, the stage of their menstrual cycle. Physical examination reveals a tachycardia and occasionally **cannon waves** may be seen in the jugular venous pulse. During AVNRT the ventricles and atria are activated simultaneously so they contract at the same time. The tricuspid valve closes with ventricular systole so the right atrium is in effect a

AVNRT

The precise mechanism by which this tachycardia is mediated is not fully known. It is generally thought that there are two separate inputs into the AV node referred to as **fast** and **slow pathways**. Each has a different rate of conduction and a different refractory period. Paradoxically, it is often the slow pathway that has the shorter refractory period. A critically timed extra-stimulus, such as an atrial extra-systole, may find one pathway refractory to its conduction, but be propagated by the other. The usual situation is for the fast pathway to be refractory and the slow pathway to be able to conduct. By the time the impulse has passed out of the slow pathway, the fast pathway is no longer refractory and is able to conduct the impulse **retrogradely** (backwards) to the atria. The sequence is then repeated and a circuit is established around the AV node. As well as each impulse conducting back to the atria, it also passes down the His Purkinje system. Thus, the ventricles are activated each time there is a circuit around the AV node and a narrow complex tachycardia ensues.

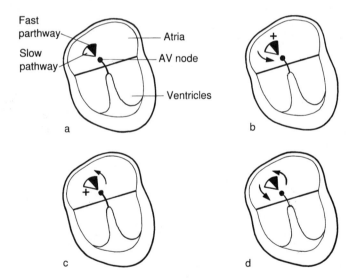

Fig. 6.4 (a) Normal. Impulse travels through the AV node from atria to ventricles. (b) In AVNRT there is an extra pathway within the AV node. An atrial extrasystole finds one pathway refractory but the other is able to conduct. (c) The pathway that was originally refractory can now conduct the impulse retrogradely (backwards) from the ventricles to atria. (d) A circuit is established around the AV node in which impulses travel forward (antegradely) through one pathway and backwards (retrogradely) through another. Each time the circuit is complete the ventricles are activated, causing a narrow complex tachycardia.

closed chamber. As it contracts right atrial pressure rises, producing striking pulsations in the neck veins called cannon waves.

The ECG usually shows a narrow QRS complex tachycardia with a rate of 150–220 beats/min. Atrial and ventricular activation are simultaneous so the P waves are 'swallowed up' in the QRS complex and are usually not seen (Fig. 6.5). Occasionally, however, the terminal part of the QRS complex is deformed by the terminal part of the P wave and this may give a clue to the diagnosis.

Treatment of the acute attack requires modification of conduction within the fast or slow pathways. Vagal stimuli (such as carotid sinus massage or Valsalva manoeuvre) may terminate the acute attack and many patients learn to do this themselves. If these are unsuccessful then verapamil or adenosine, given intravenously, almost always terminates tachycardia.

If patients are rarely troubled by attacks then prophylactic measures are not required. However, if frequent tachycardias become troublesome then consideration should be given either to prophylactic drug therapy or to cure with radiofrequency modification of the AV node. Drugs worth trying include class 1a and 1c agents (see page 123), verapamil, diltiazem and β-blockers. However, selection is largely a matter of trial and error and treatment is often imperfect. For these reasons **catheter ablation** of the slow pathway using radiofrequency energy may be performed. This prevents tachycardia without altering conduction through the AV node itself. The procedure requires a high level of expertise and is available

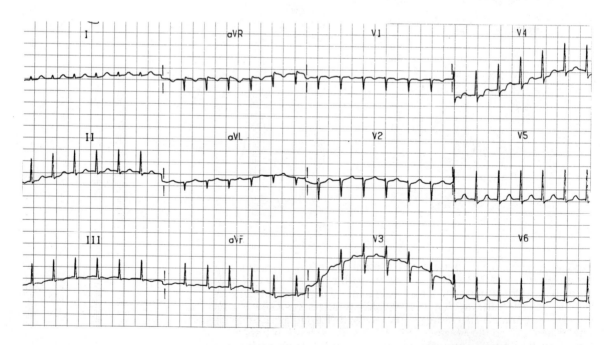

Fig. 6.5 ECG of AVNRT showing a narrow QRS complex tachycardia at a rate of 150/min. and no P waves.

only in a few specialist centres. Furthermore there is a small risk of damaging the AV node. This may create heart block and require implantation of a permanent pacemaker. Nevertheless it is likely that this technique will supercede drug therapy in years to come.

> ## Tachycardias and radiofrequency catheter ablation
>
> This technique involves the controlled destruction of the parts of the conduction system responsible for generating the tachycardia. A series of wires (rather like pacing wires) are placed in various positions throughout the heart. Careful study of the timing of the deflections recorded by these wires allows the area of abnormal tissue to be located. The wires can then be connected to a radiofrequency generator which 'burns' an area of myocardium near the tip of the wire, thereby destroying the part of the conduction system responsible for generating tachycardia. Using this technique it is possible to destroy (**'ablate'**) the accessory pathways of patients with WPW syndrome or modify the slow AV nodal pathway of patients with AVNRT. It can also be used in patients with AF when the ventricular rate cannot be controlled with drugs. In these circumstances the AV node is destroyed with subsequent insertion of a permanent pacemaker to ensure an adequate ventricular rate.

Atrio-ventricular re-entrant tachycardia

Atrio-ventricular re-entrant tachycardia (AVRT) is a slightly less common cause of paroxysmal supraventricular tachycardia than AVNRT. It is distinguished by the presence of a **direct** electrical connection between the atrium and the ventricle, *independent* of the AV node. The commonest cause of AVRT is the **Wolff–Parkinson–White syndrome** (Fig. 6.6).

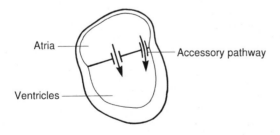

Fig. 6.6 Wolff–Parkinson–White syndrome. There is an extra (accessory) pathway connecting the atria and the ventricles. This pathway conducts faster than the AV node, so while the impulse is still in the node, the area of ventricle where the accessory pathway plugs in has already started depolarizing. It therefore has a 'head start' on normal depolarization and that portion of ventricle is said to be 'pre-excited'.

Patients with AVRT present in an identical fashion to those with AVNRT. The ECG during tachycardia usually shows narrow QRS complexes (<0.12 s, three small squares). The atria are activated

> ## AVRT
>
> Patients with this mechanism of tachycardia have an extra electrical connection between the atria and the ventricles called an **accessory pathway**. Such pathways can usually conduct both **antegradely** (forwards from atrium to ventricle) and **retrogradely** (backwards from ventricle to atrium). An impulse travelling down an accessory pathway is not delayed in the same way as an impulse conducted through the AV node. Thus the ventricles have a 'head start' in depolarization, *before* they are activated via the His Purkinje system. This early depolarization is called **pre-excitation** and produces characteristic features on the ECG in sinus rhythm. Because AV nodal delay is bypassed by conduction through the accessory pathway the **PR interval is short**. Ventricular activation by the accessory pathway occurs earlier than activation by the His Purkinje system so the QRS complex 'takes off' earlier and becomes slightly widened. This early depolarization 'slurs into' the rest of the QRS complex. The slurred part of the QRS complex is called a **delta wave** (Fig. 6.7).

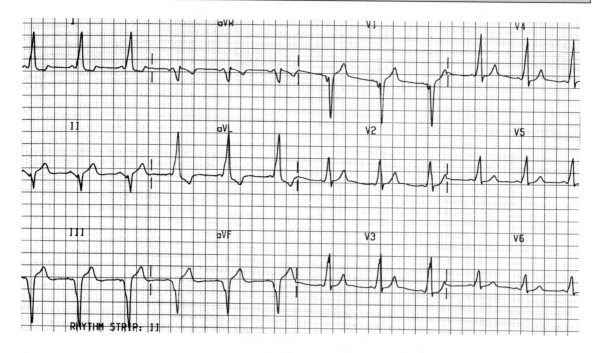

Fig. 6.7 ECG of Wolff–Parkinson–White syndrome. Note the short P–R interval (0.08 s) and the delta waves.

The mechanism of tachycardia is similar to that of AVNRT. A critically timed atrial ectopic beat may find the accessory pathway in its refractory period, but the AV node is able to conduct the impulse to the ventricle. Once through the AV node the impulse passes through the His Purkinje system to the ventricles and then backwards up the accessory pathway which is no longer refractory. Thus a rapidly conducting circuit is formed involving atria, AV node, ventricle, accessory pathway, atria, etc. the process repeating itself to cause a **re-entrant tachycardia**. The QRS complex during tachycardia is usually narrow as ventricular activation is via the normal AV node–His Purkinje route (Fig. 6.8a). This is called **orthodromic tachycardia**. Occasionally the circuit is established in reverse when the atrial ectopic is conducted *forwards* down the **accessory pathway** and *backwards* through the **AV node**. Under these circumstances ventricular activation does not take place via the usual His Purkinje system and the resulting QRS complex is broad (Fig. 6.8b). This is called **antedromic tachycardia**. Sometimes patients with Wolff–Parkinson–White syndrome may develop atrial fibrillation. In normal people the ventricles are, to a certain extent, 'protected' from very fast rates by the AV node, but if the refractory period of the accessory pathway is very short, then atrial fibrillation is conducted rapidly to the ventricles. Rarely, this may produce a dangerously rapid ventricular rate and may even result in ventricular fibrillation and death.

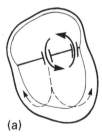
(a)

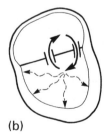
(b)

Fig. 6.8 (a) The mechanism of tachycardia in Wolff–Parkinson–White syndrome is similar to the AVNRT. In orthodromic tachycardia, impulses travel forwards through the AV node and backwards up the accessory pathway. The QRS complex is therefore narrow as ventricular activation is via the normal pathways. (b) In antedromic tachycardia, impulses travel forwards through the accessory pathway and backwards up the AV node. The QRS complexes are therefore broad as ventricular activation is not via the normal pathways.

retrogradely so sometimes P waves may be identified buried in the ST-segment or in the terminal part of the QRS complex. Atrial fibrillation with forward conduction through the accessory pathway (**pre-excited AF**) causes an irregular broad complex rhythm that is frequently mistaken for ventricular tachycardia.

Like AVNRT treatment of the acute attack is with **vagal manoeuvres**, **adenosine** or **verapamil** which alter conduction in the AV node and therefore interrupt the circuit. Occasionally drugs that block conduction in accessory pathway tissue may be useful, such as intravenous **flecainide**. Pre-excited AF requires flecainide or **DC cardioversion** (if the patient is shocked) but *never* adenosine or verapamil. These drugs block the AV node, so conduction down the accessory pathway will be favoured (**potentiated**), causing dangerous accelerations of the ventricular rate.

Prophylactic therapy follows the same principles as the treatment of AVNRT. Class 1a and 1c drugs are more useful than AV node blocking drugs in this situation. Again catheter ablation of the accessory pathway offers the chance of cure and will play an increasingly important role in the future.

Case history

A 28-year-old man became unwell during his wedding reception. He had suffered occasional palpitations for several years but they had not bothered him particularly and he had not sought medical advice. Following two glasses of champagne he became aware of his heart racing. He felt dizzy and unwell and was only just able to finish his speech. He left the reception early and missed the flight to his honeymoon in order to attend Casualty, where a 12-lead ECG showed a narrow complex tachycardia at a rate of 180 beats/min. No P waves were seen.

This is a history typical of either AVNRT or AVRT (such as Wolff–Parkinson–White). It is important to try vagal manoeuvres, such as carotid sinus massage or Valsalva, before resorting to chemical or electrical cardioversion. Possible drugs for chemical cardioversion include adenosine or verapamil, given intravenously. Once sinus rhythm is restored it is imperative to perform another ECG to look for evidence of pre-excitation (δ waves) that would be diagnostic of WPW.

Anti-arrhythmic drugs

Drugs that suppress abnormal cardiac rhythms are called **anti-arrhythmic drugs**. They act by a variety of mechanisms, although there is only a weak correlation between the type of arrhythmia and the mechanism of action of anti-arrhythmic drugs used for that particular rhythm disturbance. Hence a given arrhythmia may respond to more than one type of drug. **Vaughan Williams** classified anti-arrhythmic drugs on the basis of their mode of action and this system is widely used.

Class I drugs
These act like local anaesthetics in that they inhibit the fast inward movement of sodium ions, thereby slowing the rate of rise of the first part of the action potential. This makes cells 'less excitable' and discourages arrhythmias. Class I agents are further divided on the basis of their effect on the overall duration of the action potential.

Class Ia Prolong the action potential. Examples are **quinidine** and **disopyramide**.

Class Ib No effect on action potential duration. Examples are **lignocaine** and **mexiletene**.

Class Ic Shorten action potential. An example is **flecainide**.

Class II drugs
These are β**-blockers**. It is not clear exactly how these drugs prevent arrhythmias, but it is probably by an overall 'damping down' of the sympathetic nervous system, thereby making cells less excitable.

Class III drugs
These act by **prolonging the action potential duration**, thereby decreasing the time when cells are capable of being stimulated and generating arrhythmias. Examples include **amiodarone** and **sotalol**, the latter also having a β-blocking action.

Class IV drugs
These are **calcium antagonists** and inhibit the influx of calcium into myocardial cells. Calcium contributes more to the action potential in supraventricular tissue than ventricular tissue. Hence class IV agents (such as **verapamil**) are used for supraventricular tachycardias.

   This classification system finds no place for **digoxin** or **adenosine**. Digoxin does not prevent arrhythmias but, by increasing vagal tone, slows conduction through the AV node and reduces the number of impulses reaching the ventricle. Adenosine is a potent AV nodal blocking agent and is used for terminating tachycardia in patients with AVNRT or AVRT. It has a very short half-life and must be given by fast intravenous injection followed by a rapid saline flush.

   It should be remembered that all anti-arrhythmic drugs can themselves cause or worsen arrhythmias. This is called a **pro-arrhythmic effect** and demands that therapy should be closely monitored after careful documentation of the nature of the rhythm disturbance.

Ventricular arrhythmias

Ventricular arrhythmias arise from the ventricle. Activation of the remainder of the ventricular muscle is not via the His Purkinje system but by slow, inefficient pathways, so the hallmark of a ventricular beat is an abnormally broad QRS (greater than 0.12 s, three small squares). The rhythm disturbances produced by abnormal ventricular depolarizations are extremely variable.

Ventricular ectopics

Extra ventricular beats that interrupt normal sinus rhythm are called **ventricular ectopic beats** or **ventricular extrasystoles** (Fig. 6.9). They are usually benign and asymptomatic, but may also be a marker of underlying cardiac disease. Occasionally they cause palpitations and if these become intolerable then treatment involves removal of any of the known exacerbating factors, such as smoking and excess caffeine.

Ventricular tachycardia

If three or more ventricular beats occur together in sequence at a rate of greater than 100/min the term **ventricular tachycardia (VT)** is used. This is always pathological and is an important cause of sudden cardiac death. Ventricular tachycardia is usually due to underlying cardiac pathology, the most common cause being ischaemic heart disease. Other causes include **cardiomyopathy**, **valvular heart disease** and **congenital disorders**, but it can rarely occur in the structurally normal heart. The presenting features are variable and to an extent depend on the rate of the tachycardia and the degree of underlying cardiac dysfunction. Some patients may be asymptomatic, especially if the tachycardia is short lived, but most present with one or more of palpitation, dyspnoea, chest pain, dizziness or syncope. It is not uncommon for patients with VT to present with sudden haemodynamic collapse or even cardiac arrest. This may occur because the rapid, inefficient ventricular contractions are unable to maintain an adequate circulation, or alternatively because ventricular tachycardia degenerates into ventricular fibrillation, in which there is incoordinate electrical and mechanical activity of the heart.

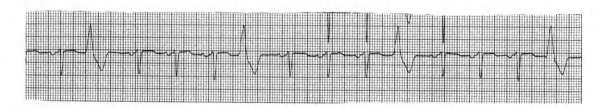

Fig. 6.9   Ventricular ectopics.

Physical examination during an attack usually demonstrates a rapid, weak pulse, often with a low blood pressure and signs of reduced cardiac output such as sweating and cool peripheries. These features are, however, non-specific so the diagnosis of VT is made chiefly from the ECG. If there is impairment of conduction through the His Purkinje system than a supraventricular tachycardia with bundle branch block will also produce a broad complex tachycardia so certain ECG features must be looked for in order to confirm the diagnosis of VT.

AV dissociation

The majority (75%) of AV nodes are unable to conduct ventricular impulses retrogradely, so activity of the sinus node and atria continue independent of ventricular activity. This is called **AV dissociation** and careful examination of the 12-lead ECG may reveal independent P waves. Sometimes atrial depolarization takes place at a critical instant when the ventricles are between beats and are therefore capable of being stimulated. Conduction spreads normally through the His Purkinje system and a narrow QRS complex is seen on the ECG. This is called a **capture beat**, because the normal atrial depolarization 'captures' the ventricle at the crucial moment between beats. Similarly, an atrial depolarization may arrive at a time when the ventricle is just beginning its activation. Further spread of depolarization is by a combination of normal His Purkinje and abnormal ventricular pathways. The result is a cross between a narrow QRS complex and a ventricular beat called a **fusion beat** (Fig. 6.10).

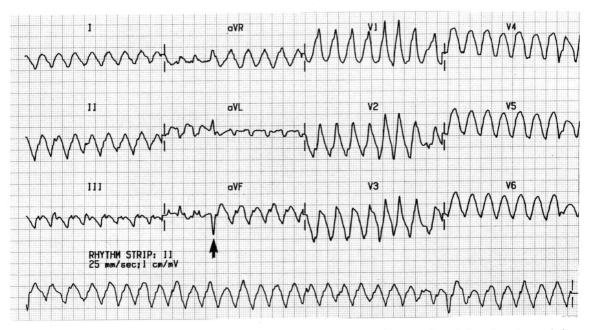

Fig. 6.10 Ventricular tachycardia. Capture and fusion beats are seen (arrowed) and there is extreme left axis deviation.

Other ECG features

When fusion and/or capture beats are present the diagnosis of VT can be made confidently. However, they are frequently not present, especially in rapid tachycardia, so other ECG features are needed in order to distinguish VT from SVT with abnormal conduction. Some of these are listed below, although they are by no means 'foolproof' and in difficult cases electrophysiological testing may be required.

ECG features that may distinguish VT from SVT with abnormal conduction

1. QRS complex greater than 0.16 s in duration
2. QRS complex showing extreme axis deviation (>30° beyond normal limits)
3. **Concordance across the chest leads**. This refers to whether the QRS complexes are similarly positive or negative in the chest leads. If they are all positive or all negative there is said to be concordance, which supports the diagnosis of VT
4. Initial positive deflection greater than second positive deflection in lead V_1 (RSr pattern)

Management of ventricular tachycardia

Even with the help of the ECG features outlined above it is often extremely difficult to distinguish VT from SVT with abnormal conduction. It is therefore good practice to treat every broad complex tachycardia as 'VT until proven otherwise' particularly for inexperienced physicians. The acute management depends largely on the patient's clinical condition. Patients who are unconscious due to cardiac arrest or a very low cardiac output should be given oxygen and **cardioverted** immediately using **DC energy**. Conscious but haemodynamically unstable patients should be **cardioverted** under a short acting **general anaesthetic**. If the patient is haemodynamically stable (adequate blood pressure and not in cardiac failure) then chemical cardioversion with intravenous **lignocaine** may be tried, but is often unsuccessful. If this is the case then other options include DC cardioversion under anaesthetic or 'overdrive pacing' the right ventricle. This involves the insertion of a pacing wire into the right ventricular apex and the delivery of stimuli at a faster rate than the tachycardia. This 'breaks the circuit' and allows the sinus node to resume its pacemaking function.

Further treatment of the acute episodes should only be given if ventricular tachycardia returns, when a lignocaine infusion may be tried. Other options in the maintenance of sinus rhythm in the acute phase include **mexiletine, disopyramide, sotalol** and **amiodarone**. Potassium levels should be measured and, if abnormal, corrected in all patients with VT.

Once the acute episode of VT has resolved management is directed towards establishing the underlying cause. **Acute** myocardial infarction (within 48 h) should be excluded, as ventricular tachycardia in this context does not require prophylactic therapy. Most patients with VT *not* due to myocardial infarction should undergo full assessment with 24-h Holter monitoring, exercise testing, echocardiography and coronary angio-graphy. Many cases of VT arise from an ischaemic or infarcted area of myocardium. If angiography shows critical coronary artery disease then the patient should be revascularized, with either angioplasty or bypass surgery. If coronary disease is not present, or thought unlikely to be causing significant ischaemia, then the patient should undergo **electrophysiological testing**. If ventricular tachycardia with a similar morphology to the presenting ECG can be induced the patient may be retested following the administration of a variety of antiarrhythmic drugs. If tachycardia is not inducible following one or more of these drugs they may be suitable for long term use as prophylaxis against ventricular arrhythmias.

Occasionally, ventricular tachycardia is inducible on exercise testing, or frequent episodes are seen on Holter monitoring. In such patients the effect of antiarrhythmic drugs in preventing tachycardia may be studied using these non-invasive methods.

The management of ventricular tachycardia has been radically altered recently by the development of the **implantable cardioverter-defibrillator (ICD)**. This is a sophisticated 'pacemaker' that continuously monitors the heart rhythm. In the event of ventricular tachycardia or fibrillation the ICD delivers a DC shock to the heart that restores sinus rhythm. This expensive therapy is suitable mainly in patients for whom no successful antiarrhythmic drug can be found. It is often the treatment of choice for patients whose initial presentation was with cardiac arrest and for whom the price of arrhythmia breakthrough on drug treatment is likely to be fatal.

Non-sustained ventricular tachycardia

If ventricular tachycardia lasts less than 30 s and terminates spontaneously it is said to be **non-sustained**. Many patients with non-sustained VT are asymptomatic. If there is no identifiable underlying cardiac pathology then treatment is usually reserved for those with symptoms. If there is underlying disease then further investigation, occasionally with electrophysiological studies to guide therapy, is indicated.

Polymorphic ventricular tachycardia

This form of ventricular tachycardia is defined as one with an unstable and continuously varying QRS morphology (Fig. 6.11). It is often seen in myocardial infarction or ischaemia and is potentially life-threatening, like any VT, due to its propensity to degenerate into ventricular fibrillation. The QRS morphology sometimes appears to twist around the isoelectric

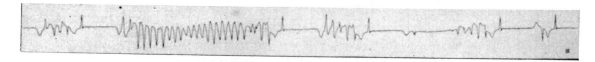

Fig. 6.11 Polymorphic ventricular tachycardia. Note the broad complex tachycardia with changing QRS axis.

baseline and is then referred to as '**torsades de pointes**' ('twisting point'). This characteristic appearance is important clinically because it is often associated with a **long QT interval** on the resting ECG. This represents prolonged ventricular repolarization and important causes include class Ia, Ic and III antiarrhythmic drugs such as **quinidine** and **amiodarone**, **psychotropic drugs** and certain **electrolyte disorders** (notably **hypocalcaemia** and **hypomagnesaemia**). It may also be a **congenital** problem. Withdrawal of the offending drug or correction of electrolyte imbalances is usually successful in acquired cases of QT prolongation. In the congenital form, β-blockers and occasionally pacing are the main of treatments.

Ventricular Fibrillation

This is the commonest cause of cardiac arrest. The electrocardiogram shows a chaotic ventricular rhythm associated with no cardiac output

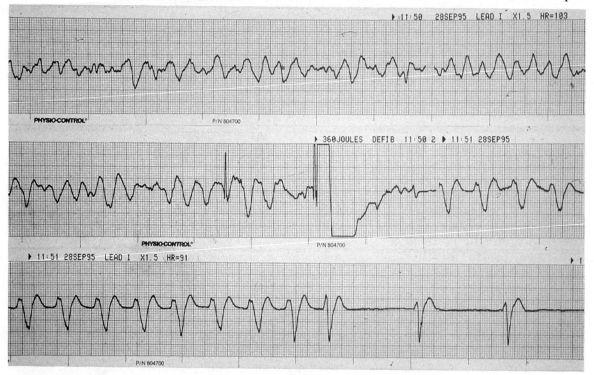

Fig. 6.12 Ventricular fibrillation. There is random incoordinate electrical activity. Atrial fibrillation follows DC cardioversion.

(Fig. 6.12). Most patients have underlying coronary artery disease and, as the arrhythmia usually occurs out of hospital, it carries a high mortality. However, prompt cardiopulmonary resuscitation and defibrillation does produce survivors and the frequency of VF in the early hours of acute myocardial infarction was the primary reason behind the development of cardiac monitoring in coronary care units, where treatment can be delivered promptly by specially trained nurses. In patients with VF not due to myocardial infarction a full investigation, similar to that described for sustained VT, is mandatory. An ICD is often the treatment of choice (if the rhythm is not due to acute myocardial infarction) as patients rarely get a second chance if ventricular fibrillation returns.

BRADYCARDIAS, DISTURBANCES OF INTRAVENTRICULAR CONDUCTION AND CARDIAC PACING

Bradycardias

A bradycardia is generally accepted as being less than 60 beats/min. As with tachycardias not all bradycardias are due to cardiac disease. When they are due to a primary cardiac disorder, they occur either as a consequence of an impairment of impulse **formation** (disease of the sinus node) or of impulse **propagation** (block in the AV node or His Purkinje system).

Sinus bradycardia

As discussed previously, the sinus node is influenced by autonomic tone. Withdrawal of sympathetic stimulation or high levels of vagal activity will slow the rate of sinus node discharge. The P waves and QRS complexes have a normal morphology, but a rate of <60/min. (Fig. 6.13). Sinus bradycardia is commonly seen in trained athletes, during sleep and with drugs such as β-blockers. Profound sinus bradycardia may occur in susceptible individuals who faint at the sight of blood or when experiencing pain. This situation is also accompanied by a fall in blood pressure and the treatment is to lie the individual down in order to encourage venous return. This results in prompt recovery in most cases but occasional patients experience frequent syncopal episodes, not always with an obvious precipitant. This is termed the **malignant vaso-vagal syndrome** and may require treatment with (paradoxically) β-blockers, disopyramide or sometimes cardiac pacing.

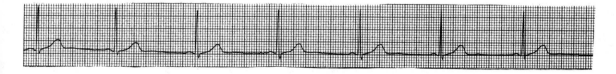

Fig. 6.13   Sinus bradycardia. Normal P waves and QRS complexes at a rate of 45/min.

Sick Sinus Syndrome

Impaired function of the sinus node is usually due either to **ischaemia** or to a poorly understood process of **fibrosis** around the cells. The sinus node may fail to generate an impulse (**sinus arrest**), may depolarize slowly (**sinus bradycardia**), or the impulses may not be conducted to the atria (**sino-atrial block**). The term 'sick sinus syndrome' is used to encompass all of these abnormalities (Fig. 6.14). The bradycardia found in such individuals justifies treatment only if it is associated with symptoms such as dizziness or syncope. Atrial or dual chamber pacing (see later) is effective in such circumstances.

If the pause between sinus beats is sufficiently long then other parts of the heart 'cut in' and take over the pacemaking. Sometimes a **tachycardia** develops after a prolonged pause, the commonest being **atrial fibrillation**. Where periods of sinus arrest or bradycardia alternate with bursts of tachycardia the term **tachy-brady syndrome** is used. Patients may get symptoms either from the tachycardias or from the pauses. Insertion of a permanent pacemaker is required to protect against bradycardias before the tachycardias can safely be treated with anti-arrhythmic drugs.

Case history

A 75-year-old man saw his GP because of recurrent dizzy episodes. On several occasions over the previous three months he had experienced a sensation of feeling as though he was about to 'black out' and on two occasions had lost consciousness for a few moments, witnessed by his wife. He denied any chest pain, shortness of breath or palpitation and was otherwise well and taking no medication. Examination was unremarkable, as was a 12-lead ECG.

This man describes symptoms of pre-syncope and syncope. 'Dizzy spells' may have a cardiovascular or a neurological cause, but in the absence of any focal neurology or history suggestive of seizures the likelihood is that these have a cardiac origin.

In this case he was referred to a cardiologist for investigation. A 24-h tape revealed numerous episodes of sinus arrest followed by bursts of atrial fibrillation (tachy-brady syndrome). Following insertion of a pacemaker his symptoms resolved completely.

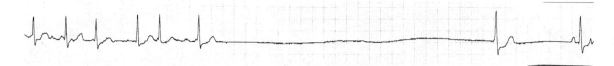

Fig. 6.14 Sick sinus. Four beats of atrial fibrillation are followed by a prolonged pause, a junctional escape beat and then a sinus beat.

Atrioventricular Block

This occurs when impulses are delayed as they pass through the AV node into the ventricles. Most cases of heart block are due to **fibrosis** of the conduction system, but other causes include **ischaemic heart disease** (especially **acute myocardial infarction**), following **cardiac surgery** and with certain **drugs** such as **digoxin**, β-**blockers** and **verapamil**. **Calcification of the aortic valve** sometimes extends into the conduction system causing heart block. It may also occur as an isolated congenital lesion. Three grades (or degrees) of AV block are recognized.

First degree AV block is defined on the electrocardiogram as a P–R interval greater than 0.2 s (five small squares) (Fig. 6.15). It requires no treatment and may be seen in fit individuals with high degrees of vagal tone.

Second degree AV block is subdivided into Mobitz Types I and II. In **Mobitz I** (also called **Wenckebach block** or **Wenckebach phenomenon**) there is progressive lengthening of the P–R interval until eventually an impulse is completely blocked (Fig. 6.16). This type of heart block may be due to high levels of vagal tone and may occur during sleep. The site of conduction block is **within the AV node** and usually no intervention is required unless the patient is symptomatic. If it occurs with symptoms then any potentially offending drugs (such as β-blockers or verapamil) should be withdrawn. If symptoms persist then consideration may be given to permanent pacing.

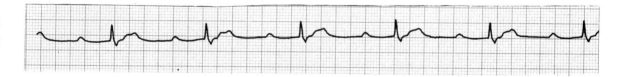

Fig. 6.15 First degree heart block. The P–R interval is prolonged at 0.44 s.

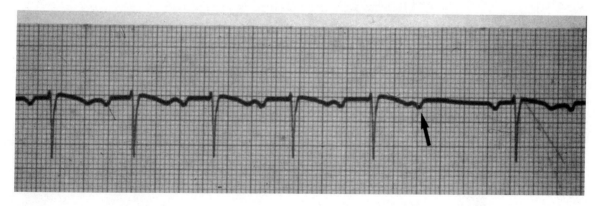

Fig. 6.16 Wenckebach (Mobitz I) second degree heart block. There is progressive lengthening of the P–R interval until eventually a P wave is not conducted (arrowed).

In **Mobitz Type II AV block** there is impaired conduction in the His Purkinje system. The P–R interval remains constant but there is intermittent non-conduction of an atrial impulse. The ECG shows several normally conducted P waves followed by a P wave on its own that has failed to 'get through' (Fig. 6.17). This form of heart block is more sinister than Mobitz I as it is more likely to progress to complete heart block. Implantation of a permanent pacemaker is indicated irrespective of symptoms.

Sometimes there is a pattern to the blockade of atrial impulses with, for example, every third or fourth P wave being non-conducted. This is an advanced form of Mobitz II and is often simply referred to as 3 : 1, 4 : 1 block, etc.

In **third degree AV block (complete heart block)** there is total failure of conduction through the AV node and none of the P waves get through. Sinus node activity continues normally so P waves can be seen at regular intervals on the ECG (Fig. 6.18). A focus below the AV node takes over as the pacemaker of the heart and dictates the ventricular rate. If the focus lies high up in the His Purkinje system then ventricular activation is via the normal electrical pathways and the QRS complex is narrow. A pacemaking focus in the myocardium causes depolarization through slow inefficient pathways and the QRS complex is wide. The ECG in complete heart block shows P waves and QRS complexes that are totally separate, reflecting completely independent activity of the atria and ventricles. This is called **AV dissociation**.

Third degree heart block is generally associated with symptoms and, because the ventricular escape rhythm is unreliable, should always be treated by **permanent pacing**. An exception is when third degree block

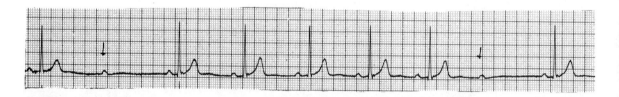

Fig. 6.17 Mobitz II second degree heart block. There is intermittent failure to conduct a P wave (arrowed), but the P–R interval is constant for conducted beats.

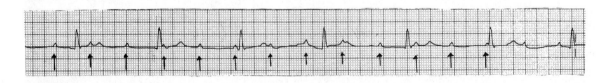

Fig. 6.18 Complete heart block. The P wave rate is regular (arrowed), but they bear no relation to the QRS complexes.

is due to inferior myocardial infarction. AV conduction usually recovers in these circumstances and management should initially be conservative.

Disturbances of Intraventricular Conduction

After an impulse exits from the AV node it travels through the His Purkinje system, initiating uniform depolarization of the ventricles. Damage to the His Purkinje system therefore impairs conduction of impulses to the ventricles. Either the right or left bundle branches may be damaged. Subsequent ventricular activation is through abnormally slow pathways so the **QRS complexes in bundle branch block are wide** and have characteristic shapes. Damage may occur more distally in the anterior or posterior fascicles of the left bundle which, again, produces characteristic ECG appearances.

Right bundle branch block (RBBB)

As discussed in Chapter 2 the left bundle is activated fractionally earlier than the right so normal activation of the interventricular septum is from **left to right**. Damage to the right bundle therefore has no effect on the direction of septal depolarization, so the initial deflections registered in leads V_1 and V_6 are normal in RBBB (small positive deflection in V_1 as the septum depolarizes towards this lead and small negative in V_6 as depolarization is away from this lead). Following septal depolarization, activation of the left ventricle proceeds normally via the left bundle but right ventricular activation is delayed due to failure of conduction through the right bundle. The chest leads record the effect of LV depolarization that is completely unopposed by right ventricular forces. V_1 (overlying the RV) registers a negative deflection and V_6 (overlying the LV) records a positive deflection. In the absence of a functioning right bundle the right ventricle is depolarized by impulses that have had to arrive via abnormal slow pathways. Hence by the time right ventricular activation takes place it does so unopposed by the left ventricle which has already completed its depolarization. V_1 records a second positive deflection and V_6 registers a negative deflection. It can be seen that lead V_1 records two positive deflections which gives the QRS complex an M shape. The first of these is smaller and is termed the r wave. The second, larger, deflection is called the R wave. Hence V_1 registers an rSR complex. This and the other ECG features of RBBB are shown in Figs 6.19 and 6.20.

Right bundle branch block may occur in normal individuals but is also seen in patients with **atrial septal defects**, with conditions that cause increased strain on the right ventricle (such as **pulmonary embolism**) and in ischaemic heart disease.

Left bundle branch block (LBBB)

Depolarization of the septum is usually from left to right via the left bundle branch. If this is damaged then septal depolarization has to be

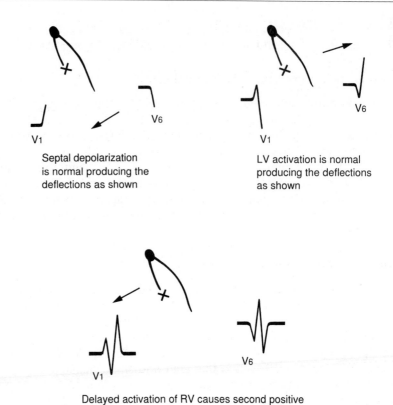

Septal depolarization
is normal producing the
deflections as shown

LV activation is normal
producing the deflections
as shown

Delayed activation of RV causes second positive
deflection in V1 and second negative deflection in V6

Fig. 6.19 Right bundle branch block. The QRS complexes are widened and there is an RSr pattern in V_1 with a deep slurred S wave in lead I.

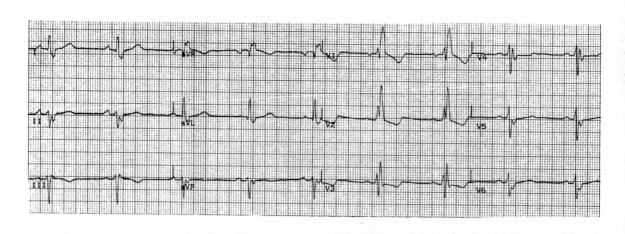

Fig. 6.20 Right bundle branch block. There is also left axis deviation.

> *ECG features of RBBB*
>
> 1. QRS complex greater than 0.12 s (three small squares).
> 2. rSR pattern in V_1.
> 3. Deep S wave in V_6 (delayed activation of RV causes negative deflection in the leads overlying the LV).
> 4. T wave inversion in V_1 (the RV depolarizes abnormally and so repolarizes abnormally).

from right to left. This causes a negative deflection in V_1 and a small positive deflection in V_6. Activation of the left ventricle is delayed due to disease of the left bundle but right ventricular depolarization is normal and proceeds unopposed. This registers a positive deflection in V_1 and a negative deflection in V_6. Left ventricular activation then proceeds by spread of depolarization through abnormal pathways from the right side, registering a second negative deflection in V_1 and a second positive

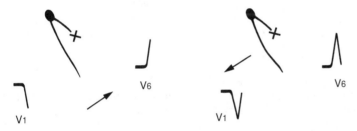

Septal depolarization is from right to left producing the deflections shown

Following septal depolarization right ventricular activation is normal producing the deflections shown

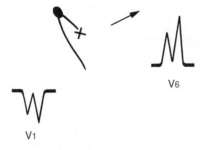

Delayed activation of the LV causes second positive deflection in V6 and a negative deflection in V1

Fig. 6.21 Left bundle branch block. The QRS complexes are widened. Note the notched ('W shaped') complexes in V_1 and the 'M shaped' complexes in V_6.

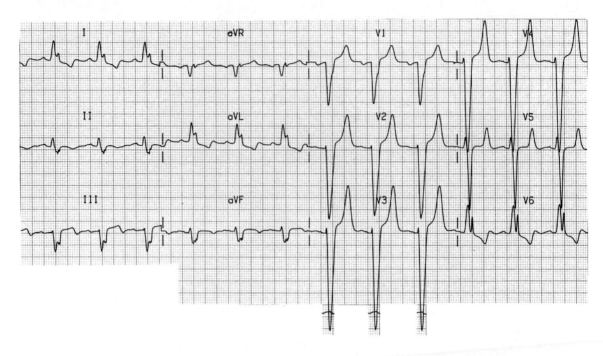

Fig. 6.22   Left bundle branch block: ECG.

deflection in V_6. Overall activation of the two ventricles takes longer than normal, so the QRS complexes are again wider than normal (Figs 6.21 and 6.22).

ECG features of LBBB

1. QRS complex greater than 0.12 s (three small squares).
2. Two negative components to QRS in V_1 (producing W shape).
3. Two positive components to QRS in V_6 (producing M shape).
4. T wave inversion in V_6 (abnormal repolarization follows abnormal depolarization).

Left anterior fascicular block (left anterior hemiblock)

The anterior fascicle of the left bundle conducts impulses to the anterosuperior aspect of the left ventricle. If this fascicle is damaged then depolarization has to spread up from the inferoposterior aspect of the left ventricle. The majority of ventricular depolarization is through the His Purkinje system so the QRS width is normal. However, because left ventricular activation is more from 'inferior to superior' the cardiac axis shifts round, resulting in **left axis deviation** on the electrocardiogram. Left anterior hemiblock can only be diagnosed when other causes of left axis deviation have been excluded (see below).

Left posterior fascicular block (left posterior hemiblock)

The posterior fascicle of the left bundle activates the inferoposterior portion of the left ventricle. Damage to this fascicle causes delayed activation of this area of myocardium. Depolarization spreads down from the anterior and superior aspect of the left ventricle, causing the cardiac axis to swing round to the right. Other causes of right axis deviation must be excluded before this finding can be attributed to block in the left posterior fascicle (see below).

Left bundle branch block and fascicular blocks generally occur in patients with underlying cardiac disease such as **coronary artery disease**, **hypertension**, **aortic stenosis** and **cardiomyopathy**. Bundle branch block in isolation does not require treatment. Sometimes different types of bundle branch block alternate and under these circumstances pacing may be indicated as the chances of progression to complete heart block are high.

Fascicular block and axis deviation

The cardiac axis is a measure of the overall direction of depolarization through the heart. Hence the axis will change if the balance of inferior, lateral and anterior ventricular forces is altered. In inferior myocardial infarction the lateral and anterior ventricular forces have more of an effect on the cardiac axis and the axis swings leftward. Left axis deviation is also seen in left ventricular hypertrophy where the increased muscle mass 'pulls the axis round' to the left. In the absence of inferior myocardial infarction or left ventricular hypertrophy, left axis deviation with a normal QRS width is due to left anterior fascicular block. By analogy, an increase in right ventricular muscle mass (right ventricular hypertrophy) or loss of lateral left ventricular muscle (due to myocardial infarction) will pull the axis round to the right. In the absence of these two pathologies right axis deviation with a normal width QRS indicates left posterior hemiblock.

Cardiac pacing

If the heart rate becomes so slow as to be insufficient for the body's requirements then it may be accelerated by the use of a **pacemaker**. These may be temporary or permanent but the underlying principle of each is the same. An electrical impulse produced by a generator is delivered to the endocardium via an electrode. Electrodes may be placed in the right atrium, right ventricle or both. The strength of the electrical impulse is sufficient to initiate depolarization and thus natural mechanical contraction of the chamber paced.

Temporary pacemakers are inserted when there is a sudden decrease in heart rate accompanied by a fall in blood pressure and symptoms such as dizziness or syncope. Following cannulation of the internal jugular or subclavian vein a pacing wire is advanced to the right ventricular apex and connected to an external pulse generator. As its name suggests this is only a temporary arrangement. It is used to 'buy time' prior to insertion of a permanent pacemaker; or in the setting of acute myocardial infarction where disturbances of conduction often resolve spontaneously.

If the rhythm disturbance is thought likely to recur then **permanent pacing** is indicated (Fig. 6.23). A variety of pacemakers are available and the choice is dictated by whether the underlying problem is one of impulse **generation** or impulse **conduction**. In **sino-atrial disease** there is an inadequate number of impulses generated due to one of the mechanisms described earlier. Those impulses that do arrive at the AV node are conducted completely normally. For patients with a 'pure' sino-atrial problem, therefore, an **atrial pacemaker** is inserted that cuts in when there is a prolonged pause between the patient's own sinus beats. Atrial contraction is triggered and the impulse is conducted normally to the ventricles. In practice, most patients with SA disease receive dual chamber pacemakers.

If the underlying problem is **AV block** then the ventricle requires pacing. Originally this involved a single electrode which detected the lack of ventricular depolarization and delivered the appropriate triggering stimulus. However, such a system is not physiological. In AV block atrial activity continues normally in spite of the lack of ventricular response. Hence it is possible that the pacemaker will activate the ventricle at the same time as the atrium contracts, producing adverse haemodynamic effects. Therefore, modern pacemakers use both atrial and ventricular electrodes. If there is AV block then the pacemaker senses when atrial contraction has occurred and delivers a ventricular stimulus after an appropriate delay. If there is co-existent sinus node disease then the atrial lead is able to 'cut in' after a prolonged sinus pause.

One important effect of sinus node disease is that the heart rate may not increase as it should during exercise. There exist very sophisticated **rate responsive pacemakers** which sense the increased body movement or respiratory rate that occurs during exercise and increase their rate of discharge appropriately.

Access to the central circulation for insertion of a permanent pacing electrode is usually via the cephalic vein. Atrial wires are manipulated into the **right atrial appendage** and ventricular wires into the **right ventricular apex**. These are connected to a pulse generator which is small enough to be buried in a pouch fashioned in front of the pectoral muscle. The whole procedure can be performed under local anaesthetic. Regular pacing checks are required and can determine when the battery within the generator is likely to wear out. Changing the generator box of a permanent pacemaker is a relatively minor procedure. Modern generators last about 10 years.

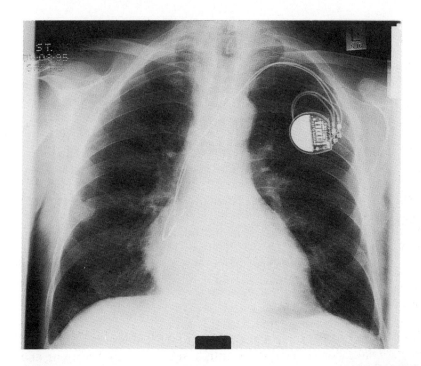

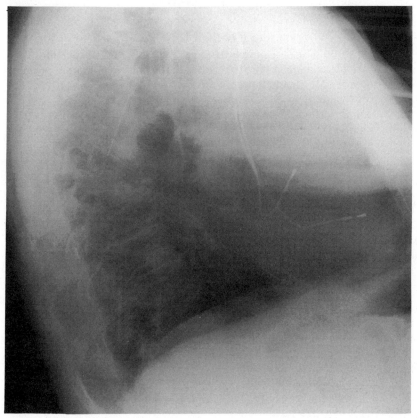

Fig. 6.23 PA and lateral chest X-rays of a patient with a permanent pacemaker. The generator box can be seen in the left pre-pectoral region and the leads are positioned in the right atrial appendage and the right ventricular apex.

CARDIAC ARREST AND RESUSCITATION

The term cardiac arrest refers to a sudden cessation in the pumping action of the heart. Victims lose consciousness within a few seconds and, unless cardiopulmonary resuscitation is commenced, death is almost inevitable. Cardiac arrest is usually due to ventricular fibrillation (in which there is random electrical activity) or asystole (in which electrical activity is absent). In some cases fast ventricular tachycardia is associated with a sufficiently low cardiac output to cause cardiac arrest.

Victims of cardiac arrest are apnoeic and pulseless. The initial aims of cardiopulmonary resuscitation (CPR; basic life support) are to ensure adequate oxygenation and cardiac output in order to avoid irreversible cerebral damage. The approach recommended by the UK Resuscitation Council is widely used.

1. **Step 1** Establish the diagnosis.
   Shake and shout at the patient to see if they are unconscious. Put a cheek near the mouth to see if they are breathing and palpate the carotid pulse.
   Call for help.
2. **Step 2** Swiftly prepare the patient for CPR. The victim should be supine and well supported (either on a bed or the floor).
   Administer a sharp praecordial thump. In some patients with VF this will restore sinus rhythm.
3. **Step 3** Commence CPR.

   A for Airway. Check the mouth for loose obstructions such as dentures, food and a 'swallowed tongue'.

   B for breathing. Gently extend the head at the atlanto-axial joint and pull the chin slightly forward (Fig. 6.24). Seal the lips round the mouth of the victim and inflate four times in quick succession.

   C for Circulation. Cardiac output is achieved by rhythmic compression of the sternum (cardiac massage). The fingers of both hands are locked together with the heel of one hand lying on the dorsum of the other. With straightened arms the lower sternum is compressed by around 2 inches and released quickly (Fig. 6.25). This produces cyclical pressure changes within the thorax and results in an adequate cardiac output. If resuscitation is performed by one person the heart is massaged at a rate of 80/min with two respirations every 15 compressions. If two people are present one respiration every five compressions at a rate of 60 compressions per minute is sufficient.

Further management (**advanced cardiac life support**; Fig. 6.26) will depend on the availability of specialized equipment and medical help. In

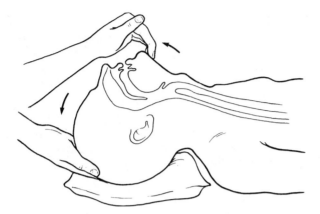

Fig. 6.24 The head is slightly extended at the atlanto-axial joint and the chin pulled slightly forward in preparation for artificial respiration in cardiac arrest.

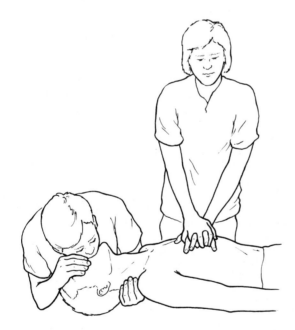

Fig. 6.25 Cardiac massage.

practice this is often what determines the order of the next steps in advance life support which include oxygen administration, defibrillation, intravenous access, ECG monitoring, intubation and intravenous cardioactive drugs. Most authorities recommend immediate defibrillation, before the underlying cardiac rhythm is established on the ECG as the chances of successful defibrillation decline with time after the onset of VF and defibrillation will do asystole no harm. Three successive shocks of

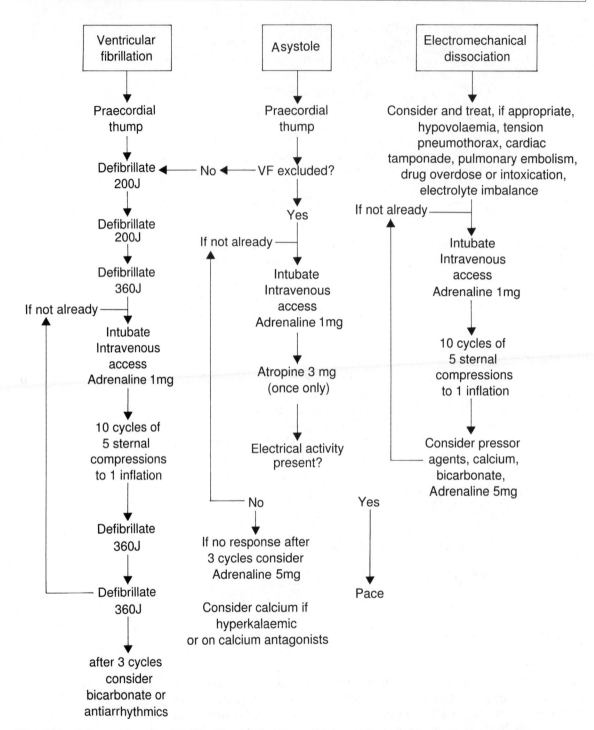

Fig. 6.26   Advanced cardiac life support (as recommended by the UK Resuscitation Council).

200, 200 and 360 Joules are given, assuming no response to the previous one. If there is still no cardiac output the rest of the above steps are carried out. At this stage patients fall into one of three groups, according to the cardiac rhythm on the ECG.

Ventricular fibrillation

If VF persists CPR should be continued and defibrillation attempted again following intravenous lignocaine. If unsuccessful adrenaline is given and defibrillation repeated. Further management is controversial, although most people try intravenous bicarbonate (acidosis makes VF more resistant) and further defibrillation. Amiodarone, bretyllium or further lignocaine may then be tried.

Asystole

Intravenous adrenaline, atropine and bicarbonate are tried in succession. Intravenous calcium may be of benefit in hyperkalaemia or in patients taking calcium channel blocking drugs such as verapamil or diltiazem.

Electromechanical dissociation

This refers to the combination of QRS complexes on the ECG but in the absence of a cardiac output. In other words there is coordinate electrical activity in the heart but no mechanical action. Important underlying causes include **cardiac tamponade**, **tension pneumothorax** and overdoses of certain drugs such as **tricyclic antidepressants**. These causes should be excluded before trying intravenous adrenaline and iso-prenaline. Calcium may be considered in hyperkalaemia or in patients taking calcium antagonists.

7 | Hypertension

PHYSIOLOGICAL BACKGROUND

With each contraction the heart pumps blood into the circulation creating the necessary pressure to drive blood across the capillary bed and ensure adequate tissue perfusion. Pressure within the arterial system is called the **blood pressure**. The level of blood pressure is determined mainly by the cardiac output and the resistance to blood flow offered by the peripheral arteries and arterioles (Fig. 7.1). These vessels have smooth muscle cells in their walls. Activation of these muscle cells causes narrowing of the vessel lumen (**vasoconstriction**). Smooth muscle relaxation causes an increase in vessel diameter (**vasodilatation**). The extent to which an artery or arteriole is constricted is called the **tone** of the vessel. Increased tone causes vasoconstriction and decreased tone causes vasodilatation. Small alterations in vessel tone produce much larger changes in peripheral resistance (and hence significant changes in blood pressure) because the resistance offered by a blood vessel depends on the cross-sectional area of

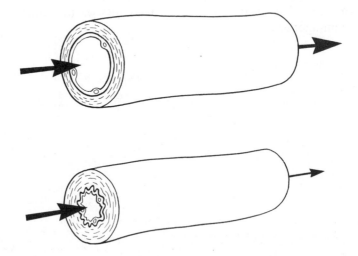

Fig. 7.1 (a) Blood flow through a dilated vessel is relatively unimpeded. (b) Resistance offered by a vessel is dependent on its cross-sectional area, so blood flow through a vasoconstricted vessel is less, unless pressure in the system increases to drive blood through.

its lumen. Arteriolar tone is regulated by a variety of vasoactive substances such as catecholamines, angiotensin and prostaglandins which act on receptors in the smooth muscle cells of the vessel. Circulating levels of these substances, in turn, are controlled by factors such as anxiety, salt and water balance and, most importantly, the **baroreceptor reflex**.

Baroreceptors

Baroreceptors are stretch receptors located in the walls of the aorta, carotid and other large arteries. High arterial pressures cause greater distension of the arterial wall which increases the activity of the baroreceptors. Afferent impulses run mainly in the vagus nerve and make central connections in the brainstem. This leads to alterations in autonomic activity which affects vascular tone and peripheral resistance. In addition connections in the hypothalamus alter the output of ACTH and vasopressin from the pituitary which in turn regulates salt and water handling by the kidney.

NORMAL AND ABNORMAL BLOOD PRESSURES

Circulatory demands are constantly changing with such factors as temperature, exercise and hormonal environment. The homeostatic mechanisms described above ensure that in most individuals blood pressure is kept within a relatively narrow range. 'Normal' blood pressure is usually defined on a statistical basis, as measurements of blood pressure in any given population have a normal (Gaussian) distribution. Hence it is possible for two individuals to have markedly different blood pressures and for them both to be within the statistical normal range. Statistics are important in blood pressure measurements because it is known that levels towards and beyond the upper end of the distribution curve are associated with increased morbidity and mortality from certain diseases such as renal failure, heart failure and stroke.

Statistical studies provide important information on the 'relative risks' of elevated blood pressure but clinical practice involves making decisions about whether to treat individual patients. It is necessary, therefore, to have some arbitrary definition of what constitutes 'hypertension'. A widely used definition of hypertension is given below and emphasizes that diastolic measurements are as important as systolic pressures when taking the decision to treat.

Grade of hypertension	Systolic pressure (mmHg)	Diastolic pressure (mmHg)
Mild	140–159	95–104
Moderate	160–179	105–114
Severe	>180	>115

CAUSES OF HYPERTENSION

In the vast majority of patients there is no obvious cause of hypertension, although it is assumed that there is some deregulation of one or more of the homeostatic mechanisms mentioned above. Such patients are said to have **primary** or **essential** hypertension. Although the precise mechanism of blood pressure elevation is not understood there are various factors that predispose to essential hypertension.

Siblings of hypertensive patients are more likely to have high blood pressure than the general population suggesting an **hereditary predisposition**. The genetic basis for this is not understood but it may involve variations (polymorphisms) in the genes that govern salt and water handling, such as the renin–angiotensin–aldosterone axis.

Immigrants to a country gradually assume the relative risk of developing hypertension as the indigenous population, suggesting that **environmental factors** are also important. Possible candidates include smoking, obesity, exercise and dietary intake of sodium. A variety of **drugs** are known to exacerbate or predispose to hypertension and do so by one of two mechanisms. **Salt and water retention** may be caused by steroids (either glucocorticoids or oestrogens in the contraceptive pill) or non-steroidal anti-inflammatory drugs (NSAIDs). Drugs which cause hypertension by **vasoconstriction** include monoamine oxidase inhibitors (MAOIs) and certain recreational drugs such as 'ecstasy'.

In a few patients there is an identifiable cause of the elevated blood pressure. This is called **secondary hypertension** and is more common in younger patients with hypertension. It is important to identify such cases as therapy (either surgical or medical) is directed at the underlying cause.

Certain **endocrine disorders** cause hypertension. In **Cushing's** and **Conn's** syndromes increased levels of glucocorticoid and mineralocorticoid, respectively, cause hypertension by salt and water retention. In **phaeochromocytoma** increased catecholamine secretion causes hypertension by α-adrenoceptor-mediated vasoconstriction. The mechanism of hypertension in **acromegaly** is not understood.

Coarctation of the aorta is a congenital cardiac defect in which there is a narrowing of the aorta beyond the origin of the vessels to the arms and head. As a result renal perfusion is poor and activation of the renin angiotensin system causes salt and water retention. Hypertension in the upper limbs (proximal to the stenosis) is marked but blood pressure in the lower limbs (distal to the aortic narrowing) is low.

Most secondary hypertension is due to **renal disease**. Disorders of either the vasculature or the parenchyma may be responsible. **Glomerulonephritis**, either acute or chronic, may cause hypertension, probably by salt and water retention. Other causes include connective tissue disorders such as systemic lupus and polyarteritis nodosa and polycystic kidney disease. In **renal artery stenosis** (Fig. 7.2) renal perfusion is impaired, due either to an **atheromatous lesion** (generally in older patients) or to proliferation of the muscular layer of the artery (this is called **fibromuscular dysplasia** and is more common in younger

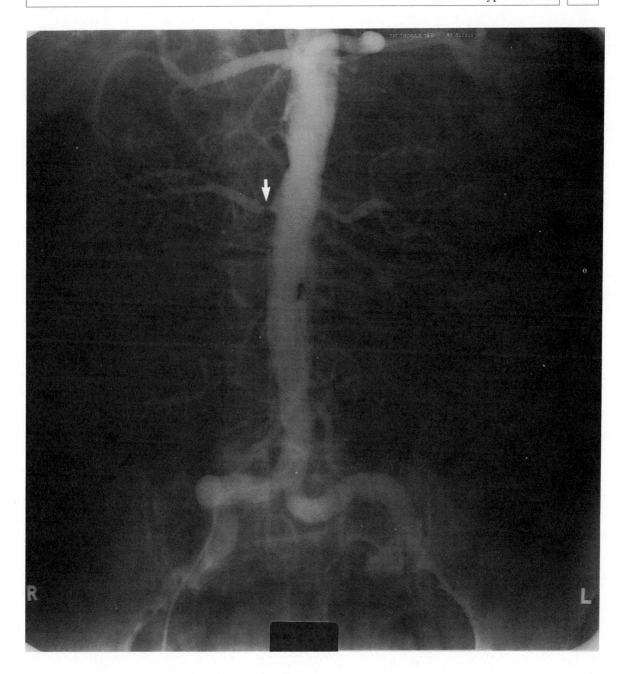

Fig. 7.2 Angiogram of renal artery stenosis. Note the narrowing (arrowed) in the proximal portion of the right renal artery.

patients). Activation of the renin-angiotensin system results in hypertension. It is often difficult to distinguish between renal disease causing hypertension and hypertension leading to renal damage.

EFFECTS OF HYPERTENSION

Morbidity and mortality amongst hypertensive patients is higher than in normotensive individuals. This is because high blood pressures damage a variety of organs, most notably **brain**, **kidney**, **heart** and **eyes**.

Hypertension increases the resistance against which the left ventricle must contract and the LV undergoes compensatory **hypertrophy** in order to maintain cardiac output. A new 'steady state' is established in which peripheral resistance to cardiac emptying is high but the heart is able to compensate for this by the thicker LV wall and the patient remains asymptomatic. With time the LV is unable to overcome this increased afterload and **heart failure** supervenes. Hypertension is also a risk factor for the development of **coronary artery disease** and is additive to factors such as smoking and diabetes in this respect.

Increased pressure in the cerebral blood vessels predisposes to the formation of **microaneurysms**, particularly in the lenticulostriate arteries around the basal ganglia and midbrain. These may rupture, causing **haemorrhagic stroke**. Hypertension is also a risk factor for the development of atheromatous lesions in the carotid and vertebral vessels.

Hypertension causes the renal vasculature to undergo various changes. The intima thickens and hardens, so that the delicate homeostatic mechanisms that govern renal perfusion are disrupted. Glomerular filtration falls off, leading to worsening hypertension as renin–angiotensin activation with salt and water retention is triggered. There is usually some impairment of tubular and excretory function, but this is less marked than in conditions such as chronic glomerulonephritis.

The changes in the blood vessels of the eyes as a result of hypertension are discussed below.

CLINICAL ASSESSMENT OF A PATIENT WITH HYPERTENSION

Most hypertensive patients are asymptomatic and are discovered on routine examination. A few people present with nose bleeds but, contrary to popular belief, headaches are rare unless there is accelerated hypertension with cerebral oedema (see below). When assessing a patient with hypertension three questions must be considered:

1. Is the patient truly hypertensive?
2. Is there an underlying cause for the hypertension?
3. Is there any evidence of end-organ damage?

It is important to ask about previous documented hypertension or normotension, symptoms of endocrine disease and to take a full drug history, especially concerning the use of **steroids** and the **contraceptive pill**. A family history of elevated blood pressure supports the diagnosis of essential hypertension. A dietary history including alcohol and salt intake is imperative as they provide the focus for non-pharmacological treatment measures. Symptoms of angina, heart failure or previous stroke suggest that significant end-organ damage has occurred.

The principles and technique of measuring blood pressure are described in Chapter 1. It is not unusual for the stress of a medical examination to give spuriously high blood pressure readings, so before labelling someone as being hypertensive it is usual practice to measure the blood pressure on three or four separate occasions over the course of several weeks, with an adequate period of rest before each reading. If it is felt that anxiety is repeatedly giving rise to falsely high readings then **ambulatory monitoring** may be used. This involves the patient wearing a blood pressure cuff for a full 24 h. An attached machine records the blood pressure at various intervals throughout the day giving a more accurate idea of whether the patient is truly hypertensive.

The remainder of the examination aims to answer the above questions. Truncal obesity, thin skin, striae and hirsutism are characteristic features of Cushing's syndrome. Patients with coarctation have weak, delayed femoral pulses with a continuous murmur heard between the scapulae (Chapter 8). A bruit may be heard in renal artery stenosis. Patients with chronic renal failure may look unwell with a sallow complexion.

Clinical evidence for end-organ damage comes from examination of the cardiovascular system, optic fundi and urinalysis. High pressures in the proximal aorta at the end of systole close the aortic valve with increased force. This may be heard as a **loud second heart sound**. As the LV hypertrophies its relaxation properties change. The LV wall becomes stiff so that efficient diastolic filling is impaired. The left atrium contracts with increased force at the end of diastole in order to force blood into the LV and improve cardiac output. This may produce a **fourth heart sound** just before S_1 and the onset of ventricular systole. The **apex beat** may be **forceful** in character due to the increased ventricular mass. If LV failure supervenes, the ventricle dilates and the **apex** is **displaced** inferolaterally and becomes more diffuse and dyscoordinate. Occasionally longstanding hypertension leads to incompetence of the aortic valve and the characteristic **early diastolic murmur** heard after the second heart sound.

Vascular changes in the eye may be visualized with an ophthalmoscope. Four grades are recognized:

1. **Narrowed tortuous arteries**. The arterial walls become thickened which increases the amount of light they reflect. This causes a characteristic appearance called **silver wiring**.
2. **AV Nipping**. This refers to the tapered appearance of veins where they cross arteries and is caused by the thickened arterial wall pressing on veins at cross-over points.
3. **Cotton wool spots** are fluffy white areas that represent the oedema that accompanies microinfarcts of the retina. High blood pressure leads to damage in the vessel wall with subsequent narrowing of the lumen and an impaired retinal blood supply. If the wall of the vessel

is breached then there is **haemorrhage** into the retina. These are characteristically **flame shaped**.

4. **Papilloedema**. This is swelling of the optic disc and in the context of hypertension occurs when there is loss of autoregulation of cerebral blood flow with brain oedema.

Stages 3 and 4 suggest that there has been significant damage to the vessel wall as a result of hypertension and urgent treatment is mandatory. If there is significant renal damage there may be proteinuria and/or haematuria on dipstick testing.

INVESTIGATIONS

Again these are directed at answering the questions of whether there is an underlying cause and if there is any end-organ damage.

Tests for secondary causes of hypertension are usually only undertaken in patients under 40 or if there is a high clinical index of suspicion. Conn's syndrome is due to excessive aldosterone secretion and causes electrolyte imbalances. Aldosterone controls exchange of sodium for hydrogen or potassium in the distal tubule of the kidney, so in Conn's syndrome large amounts of potassium and hydrogen are lost in the urine resulting in alkalosis with low serum potassium levels. Cushingoid patients should be investigated appropriately with dexamethasone suppression tests and measurements of diurnal cortisol rhythm. Three separate 24-h urinary collections for catecholamines are required to exclude phaeochromocytoma. Patients with clinical evidence of coarctation require echocardiography and/or angiography. The decision to investigate for a possible renal cause of hypertension is difficult and is discussed below.

Investigating patients for renal hypertension

There are no set rules about when to investigate a patient for a renal cause of hypertension. Clinically an abdominal or renal bruit may suggest renal artery stenosis, but there are no other clinical features that are particularly helpful in the decision. A widely accepted approach is to investigate:

1. patients under 40;
2. patients with drug resistant hypertension;
3. malignant hypertension;
4. patients with hypertension and any evidence of abnormal renal function such as raised urea/creatinine or protein/blood on dipstick testing.

A number of investigations may be used in defining renovascular causes of hypertension. Ultrasound scanning identifies renal size and abnormal structure such as polycystic disease. A difference in length of the two kidneys of 1.5 cm or more suggests a local pathology such as unilateral renal artery stenosis. Bilaterally small kidneys (less than 9 cm) suggest a pathology affecting both kidneys such as chronic glomerulonephritis. **Isotope scans** give information regarding kidney function. ^{131}I-labelled **hippuran** is injected into a vein and gamma counters placed over both kidneys. There is reduced perfusion of the kidneys supplied by the stenosed artery so less radioactivity is detected on that side. Used together these techniques detect almost all cases of renovascular hypertension, although they cannot predict whether blood pressure will respond to correction of the abnormality. **Renal angiography** is the gold standard for identifying the anatomy of the renal vessels, but does not provide information about the functional significance of stenotic lesions and is invasive.

Investigations that assess end-organ damage focus on the heart and kidney. A biochemical screen documents the plasma potassium prior to starting diuretic therapy and is a good screen for Conn's syndrome (see above). Elevated urea and creatinine provide evidence of any gross renal dysfunction. Urine dipstick testing identifies proteinuria and/or

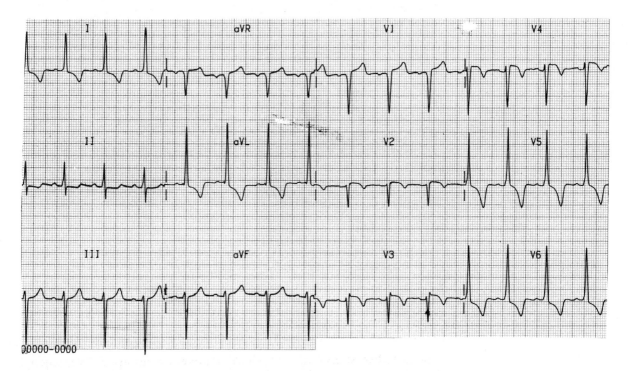

Fig. 7.3 ECG of a patient with hypertension showing increased voltage deflections and S–T depression in I, aVL, V$_5$ and V$_6$ indicating LV 'strain'.

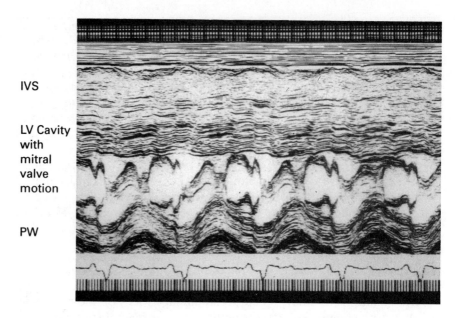

IVS

LV Cavity
with
mitral
valve
motion

PW

Fig. 7.4   Echocardiogram of a patient with longstanding hypertension. Note the thickened septum and LV wall. IVS = intersentricular septum. PW = posterior LV wall. (Both usually < 11mm thick, but in this case both are 15mm.) LV = left ventricular cavity with mitral valve motion.

haematuria. The presence of haematuria may represent an active urinary sediment (indicating an inflammatory renal disorder) or a malignant process. Both require investigation. The presence of proteinuria and/or abnormal urea and electrolytes should prompt a fuller assessment of renal function including 24-h protein excretion and creatinine clearance, together with a renal ultrasound.

Cardiac damage is assessed with a chest X-ray (which shows heart size and any cardiac failure) and an ECG which may show exaggerated voltages in the leads that examine the left ventricle indicating muscle hypertrophy. An important ECG feature sometimes seen is S–T segment depression with deep inverted T waves in the leads that overly the LV (Fig. 7.3). This represents abnormal repolarization of ventricular muscle following contraction and indicates that the ventricle is under 'strain' from the abnormally high afterload. **Echocardiography** (Fig. 7.4) identifies and can quantify LV wall thickening in hypertension but is not routinely carried out.

TREATMENT

When to treat hypertension

Hypertension is not a disease where treatment is curative. Most patients with hypertension are asymptomatic and therapy is aimed at reducing the risk of developing end-organ complications. Studies have shown a statistically significant correlation between the level of systolic blood pressure and the risk of death from cardiovascular causes. However a beneficial effect of treatment at all levels of blood pressure has been difficult to prove. There is no doubt that treatment of malignant hypertension saves lives. Untreated, 75% of these patients will die within a year; that figure falling to 30% with adequate therapy. Most doctors also agree that treatment of severe hypertension (>180 systolic; >110 diastolic) is imperative as the relative risk of cardiovascular-related death is so great. With mild elevations of blood pressure such as 150 systolic and 90–100 diastolic the potential benefit from treatment is small. An important factor in the decision of whether to treat such levels of blood pressure is the presence of other risk factors for cardiovascular disease. Smoking and hyperlipidaemia potentiate the effect of hypertension in the development of vascular disease and it is reasonable to take a more aggressive line in the treatment of mild hypertension in such 'high-risk' patients.

General measures

It is important to try non-pharmacological measures first in the treatment of hypertension. Where relevant and possible, medications that may provoke hypertension should be discontinued (such as glucocorticoids or the contraceptive pill). Obese patients should be encouraged to exercise and lose weight. Excess intake of tobacco and alcohol should be moderated. The effect of salt restriction is not proven, but diuretic therapy may be ineffectual unless dietary salt intake is reduced.

Drug therapy

Where general measures fail to restore blood pressure to a satisfactory level drugs that lower pressure (**antihypertensive agents**) are used. A variety of different drugs are available and the choice often depends on the presence of co-existent disease such as heart failure or angina.

Diuretics such as thiazides have an antihypertensive effect that is not fully understood. Certainly they cause salt loss, but more powerful diuretics such as frusemide do not have a greater antihypertensive action. Furthermore the initial salt and water loss that occurs when thiazides are started is recovered over several weeks with activation of the renin–angiotensin–aldosterone system, yet there is a sustained lowering of blood pressure. It is possible that diuretics act directly on blood vessel walls causing vasodilatation. Diuretics are particularly suitable for use if there is co-existent heart failure, when they are often used in conjunction with angiotensin-converting enzyme inhibitors (see below). They are also cheap.

β-blockers are widely used in the treatment of hypertension, particularly if the patient also has angina. Pharmacologically they antagonize the effect of endogenous catecholamines but the mechanism by which they lower blood pressure is not known. A reduction in cardiac output, resetting of the baroreceptor reflex and reduced renin activity have all been postulated.

Calcium antagonists such as nifedipine, amlodipine or verapamil are often used for hypertension. Smooth muscle cells in the walls of peripheral blood vessels are activated by intracellular calcium. Hence drugs that block the influx of calcium into smooth muscle cells lead to a lowering of the tone of the vessel wall. Vasodilatation causes peripheral resistance to fall and blood pressure is lowered.

Angiotensin-converting enzyme inhibitors (ACEIs) block the conversion of angiontensin I to angiontensin II. AT II is a powerful vasoconstrictor so ACEIs cause vasodilatation and a fall in blood pressure. These drugs are well tolerated and are particularly suitable if there is co-existent heart failure. Occasionally they cause hypotension, more commonly in patients taking diurectics. Diuretic-induced salt loss activates the renin–angiotensin–aldosterone system in an attempt to conserve body sodium. Sudden blockade of this pathway by drugs such as **captopril** and **enalapril** may cause marked vasodilatation as circulating levels of AT II fall rapidly.

There are a number of other, older antihypertensive agents available, most of which act by causing vasodilatation. Some such as **prazosin**, antagonize the action of endogenous catecholamines at α-receptors on smooth muscle walls. Others, such as **hydrallazine**, seem to have a direct vasodilator action on blood vessel walls.

Combination treatment

It is sensible to start treatment with a single agent and add in a second if adequate control is not achieved. Good combinations are diuretics with an ACEI as the activation of renin and angiotensin that accompanies diuretic-induced salt loss is antagonized by the ACEI. Calcium antagonists and β-blockers are often used together, particularly in patients with coronary artery disease. The vasodilatation that occurs with nifedipine sometimes causes an undesirable increase in heart rate (**reflex tachycardia**). This may worsen angina and can be prevented by the use of β-blockers.

Particular mention should be made of treating **hypertension** in **pregnancy**. The drug of choice in this situation is α-**methyl dopa**, which seems to act via a central nervous system effect. When urgent control of blood pressure is required intravenous **hydrallazine** is often used.

Treating secondary causes of hypertension

If there is an identifiable cause of hypertension treatment is aimed at correcting the underlying abnormality. In the case of coarctation of the aorta treatment is by surgical resection or ballooning of the narrowed segment of aorta (Chapter 8). If there is an identifiable **adrenal adenoma** causing Conn's syndrome surgical removal is the preferred treatment. In many cases, however, the cause of the elevated levels of aldosterone is not known. The choice of drug in such cases is the aldosterone antagonist **spironolactone**. Most cases of phaeochromocytoma are amenable to surgical resection. This is a hazardous operation and full blockade of α- and β-adrenoceptors is needed pre-operatively. This is achieved with **phenoxybenzamine** and **propranolol**, which block α and β receptors respectively. Renal artery stenosis may be treated surgically or with balloon angioplasty, although blood pressure may not fall following correction of the abnormality. Treatment of hypertension due to renal parenchymal disorders (such as polycystic disease and connective tissue disorders) is medical and follows similar lines to essential hypertension. Blood pressure is often difficult to control in these patients and more than one drug may be required.

Case history

A 50-year-old lady was found by the Practice Nurse to have a blood pressure of 168/116 when she attended the surgery for a routine cervical smear. She was otherwise asymptomatic and on no medication. She smoked 10 cigarettes a day. On examination she was overweight, but there was little else to find. After 15 minutes resting on the couch the blood pressure was 166/112.

This lady may be genuinely hypertensive, but the stress of attending for a cervical smear may be a contributory factor. Before labelling her as 'hypertensive' she should have her blood pressure checked at least twice more, separated by several days, with an adequate period of rest before each. If repeatedly high values are recorded then it is reasonable to conclude that she has 'moderate' hypertension. Baseline investigations to document end-organ damage include electrolytes, urinalysis, ECG and CXR. Assuming these are normal and in the absence of any clinical evidence for a secondary cause it is safe to assume she has 'essential' hypertension.

Management involves explanation about the importance of blood pressure control, advice about weight reduction, stopping smoking and regular, gentle exercise. If these general measures do not restore her blood pressure to a satisfactory level then treatment should be started.

ACCELERATED (MALIGNANT) HYPERTENSION

The term 'malignant' in this case does not refer to hypertension associated with underlying neoplasia. Rather, it is used to emphasize the dismal prognosis of this condition in which very high blood pressures (usually >140 diastolic) occur in association with severe structural damage to arterial vessel walls. It is characterized by a rapid rise in blood pressure and occurs more often in patients with an underlying cause, although it may also occur in essential hypertension. It is more common in smokers. The underlying process involves damage to the endothelium by very high arterial pressures. There is an inflammatory reaction in the media of the arterial wall which, when stained and examined under a microscope, resembles fibrin. This has led to the term **fibrinoid necrosis** which is the pathological hallmark of accelerated hypertension. The inflammatory reaction in the wall of the artery causes narrowing of the lumen. Arteries and arterioles lose their ability to autoregulate blood flow leading to rupture of capillaries with infarction and necrosis of the tissues that they supply. Clinically, the most important vessels to be affected are the cerebral, retinal and renal arteries. This explains the common clinical features of headache (due to cerebral oedema), visual disturbance and renal failure. Occasionally altered consciousness and seizures may occur with accelerated hypertension and this is called **hypertensive encephalopathy**. Left ventricular failure with pulmonary oedema is not uncommon. Echocardiography often reveals a normal LV wall thickness, suggesting that the rise in blood pressure has occurred rapidly. The LV does not have time to undergo compensatory hypertrophy in response to the rapid increase in afterload and LV failure results.

Examination may reveal a gallop rhythm and lung crepitations from heart failure; haemorrhages and exudates on the retina; papilloedema; and proteinuria on dipstick testing.

Accelerated hypertension is a medical emergency as 70% of patients will die within a year if left untreated. Cerebral arteries lose their ability

---

Case history

A 34-year-old West Indian man was found at a London Transport employment medical to be hypertensive. He was entirely asymptomatic and had no previous past medical history. His parents emigrated from Antigua in the early 1960s, but his father died shortly after arriving from a 'funny stroke' his mother said. On examination his blood pressure was 240/150, fundoscopy revealed widespread haemorrhages and exudates and there was 3+ proteinuria on dipstick testing. There was no radio-femoral delay, abdominal mass or renal bruit.

This man has malignant hypertension. The combination of very high blood pressure and retinal haemorrhages requires urgent admission to hospital for anti-hypertensive treatment and investigation for an underlying cause. These include electrolytes, urine microscopy, markers of 'autoimmune' connective tissue diseases and renal ultrasound.

In this case the underlying cause was polycystic kidney disease. This is associated with Berry aneurysms and it is possible that his father's 'funny stroke' was a subarachnoid haemorrhage from a ruptured aneurysm.

to regulate blood flow and if blood pressure is reduced too quickly cerebral perfusion may be sufficiently impaired to cause infarction and stroke. Treatment of malignant hypertension therefore involves initially cautious doses of drugs with short half-lives such as intravenous **nitroprusside** or **labetolol**. If blood pressure falls precipitously then cessation of the infusion quickly corrects this. Once the blood pressure has been controlled with intravenous drugs then maintenance oral medication may be started. All patients with malignant hypertension should undergo screening for an underlying cause.

8 | Cardiomyopathies

A cardiomyopathy is a disorder of heart muscle for which there is no readily identifiable cause. They are classified into dilated, obstructive and restrictive disorders on the basis of the nature of the cardiac dysfunction and the resultant haemodynamic abnormalities.

DILATED CARDIOMYOPATHY

This condition is characterized by dilatation and poor systolic function of both ventricles in the absence of underlying coronary artery, valvular, congenital or hypertensive heart disease. The relative proportion of right and left ventricular dysfunction is variable, although patients tend to present with symptoms of left ventricular failure. The heart becomes progressively more dilated like a 'flabby bag' and unable to empty satisfactorily during systole. A larger than normal volume of blood remains in the ventricle at the end of systole which, when added to venous return, leads to high end-diastolic pressures. In addition poor cardiac output invokes the compensatory mechanisms described in detail in Chapter 3. Activation of the renin–angiotensin system causes salt and water retention and an increase in afterload on the heart. **Sympathetic mediated vasoconstriction** redirects blood centrally in order to safeguard vital organ perfusion. The resultant increase in venous return finds a heart functioning on a flat Starling curve and unable to increase its output.

Although, strictly speaking, the cause of cardiomyopathy is unknown it is common practice to include in the 'dilated cardiomyopathy' group conditions with similar clinical features, but for which an aetiological agent is apparent. Such causative agents include alcohol, cytotoxic drugs such as adriamycin and iron overload.

Dilated cardiomyopathy

Commonest form of cardiomyopathy
Ventricular dilatation
Poor systolic function

No coronary artery disease
No valvular heart disease
No hypertensive heart disease

Clinical features

Patients usually present with symptoms of left ventricular failure, particularly fatigue and exertional dyspnoea. Oedema due to right ventricular dysfunction usually develops at some stage, but the timing of this is variable. Chest pain is infrequent. Arrhythmias, particularly atrial fibrillation, are common and may cause abrupt haemodynamic deterioration as the absence of atrial contraction reduces the efficiency

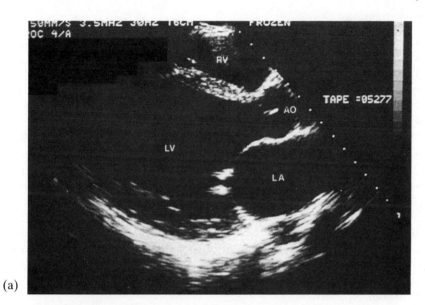

(a)

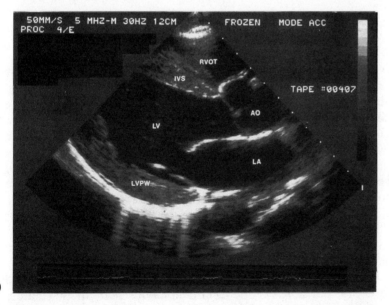

(b)

Fig. 8.1 Echocardiogram of a patient with dilated cardiomyopathy showing grossly dilated left ventricle (a), with that of a normal for comparison (b).

of diastolic filling. Ventricular arrhythmias (VT and VF) are a common cause of death in patients with dilated cardiomyopathy.

Examination reveals a **displaced apex beat** (due to ventricular dilatation) which is often rather diffuse and dyscoordinate. This may be thought of as being due to a flabby, overloaded ventricle that contracts poorly. Oedema, lung crepitations and added heart sounds are usual. Patients may be in atrial fibrillation.

Investigations

These include tests to rule out conditions with an underlying cause. Thyroid function and iron studies should be checked as correction of any abnormalities may result in clinical improvement. An ECG may show non-specific ST–T wave abnormalities or left bundle branch block and helps exclude coronary artery disease as the cause of left ventricular dysfunction. The CXR usually shows cardiomegaly and evidence of pulmonary venous congestion. Echocardiography demonstrates dilatation and poor systolic function of all four cardiac chambers (Fig. 8.1). It helps exclude a valvular cause of ventricular dysfunction, although there is often mitral and tricuspid regurgitation due to stretching of the respective valvular rings by dilated ventricles. Cardiac catheterization is not usually necessary but if performed should confirm normal coronary arteries. Myocardial biopsy rarely provides useful clinical information. Measurement of the pulmonary vascular resistance is required when assessing patients for heart transplantation as a very high resistance will result in acute right ventricular failure in the newly transplanted heart.

Dilated CMO and myocarditis

Although the precise cause of dilated cardiomyopathy is, by definition, unknown some people believe that it follows certain **viral infections**. Increased titres of Coxsackie antibodies have been noted in some patients with dilated cardiomyopathy, although their pathological significance is questionable. The hypothesis is also fuelled by the knowledge that a proportion of patients with acute viral illnesses complicated by **myocarditis** may go on to develop a dilated cardiomyopathy. Myocarditis itself is a condition that is difficult to diagnose. Non-specific ST–T wave changes are relatively common with acute viral illness but whether this represents genuine heart damage is debatable. A few patients with viral infection develop an acute 'cardiac illness' with variable amounts of heart failure and pericarditis and this is what many refer to as **acute viral myocarditis**. Most enjoy swift and complete recovery, but a few patients are left with permanent (mainly systolic) cardiac dysfunction.

Treatment

Attention should be paid to any underlying correctable aetiology. Further management includes diuretics, ACE inhibitors, digoxin and nitrates as outlined in Chapter 3. Patients with AF should be anticoagulated with warfarin. Arrhythmias other than atrial fibrillation are usually treated with amiodarone as it is the least negatively inotropic agent. **Heart transplantation** is an option in selected patients.

HYPERTROPHIC CADIOMYOPATHY

This condition is characterized by generalized myocardial hypertrophy in the absence of any obvious cause such as hypertension or aortic valve disease. The interventricular septum is usually the site of hypertrophy although the free wall and apex of the left ventricle may also be involved. The condition emphasizes how important diastole is for normal cardiac function. The hypertrophied ventricles contract with increased vigour, but they have abnormal relaxation properties and diastolic filling is impaired. The atria have to work harder in order to force blood into the ventricles and a greater filling pressure is required to maintain cardiac output. Hypertrophy of the septum may interfere with mitral valve function. The increased force of septal contraction pulls the anterior leaflet of the mitral valve forward, giving rise to mitral regurgitation. The mass of contracting hypertrophied muscle may also obstruct the left ventricular outflow tract. For this reason the condition is sometimes called **hypertrophic obstructive cardiomyopathy** (HOCM).

Classically the condition is hereditary, with an autosomal dominant trait, but sporadic cases also occur. The natural history is extremely variable. Some individuals exhibit an aggressive form of the condition with heart failure or lethal ventricular arrhythmias early. Others remain asymptomatic indefinitely.

Clinical features

Most patients present with exertional dyspnoea due mainly to high left atrial pressures, although mitral regurgitation may also contribute. Angina is not uncommon, despite normal coronary arteries, as the hypertrophied ventricles have an abnormally high oxygen demand. Arrhythmias may manifest as palpitation or, in the case of ventricular arrhythmias, sudden death. The onset of atrial fibrillation often causes an abrupt clinical deterioration as ventricular filling is worsened by the loss of atrial contraction. Occasionally the condition is diagnosed following the detection of a cardiac murmur at a routine physical examination or after a family screening programme.

The ventricle contracts forcefully and completes most of its emptying early in systole. After this the outflow tract becomes obstructed and the aortic valve closes. Consequently the **carotid pulse** often has a characteristic jerky character as most of the cardiac output is ejected over a short period of time. Strong atrial contraction just prior to ventricular systole may give the apex a 'double impulse' feel and the ventricular component of the apex beat is forceful. Vigorous atrial contraction may also be heard as a fourth heart sound. Turbulent flow through the partially obstructed outflow tract may produce a harsh systolic murmur similar to that of aortic stenosis. The murmur of mitral regurgitation may also be heard.

Investigations

These include an ECG which shows evidence of left ventricular hypertrophy and strain (Fig. 8.2) or left bundle branch block. CXR may show cardiomegaly. The definitive investigation is an echocardiogram which clearly demonstrates myocardial hypertrophy (Fig. 8.3), excludes aortic stenosis, and also identifies other features of the condition. These include movement of the mitral valve leaflets towards the interventricular septum (anteriorly) during systole, asymmetrical septal hypertrophy and premature closure of the aortic valve. Cardiac catheterization is not usually required but is sometimes performed to exclude coronary artery disease as an explanation for angina. Left ventricular angiography reveals a characteristic banana-shaped ventricle with occlusion of the cavity during systole. Measurements of pressure in the left ventricle may reveal a pressure gradient within the cavity.

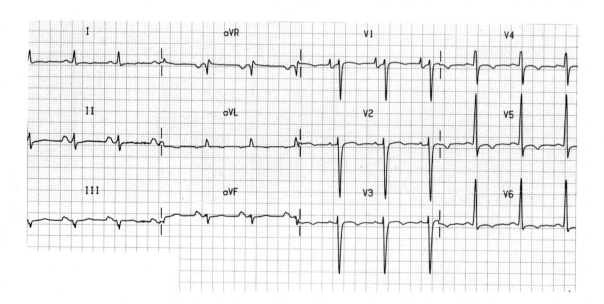

Fig. 8.2 ECG in hypertrophic cardiomyopathy often shows left ventricular hypertrophy with strain. In this ECG the biphasic P wave in V_1 indicates left atrial hypertrophy in response to the stiff non-compliant left ventricle.

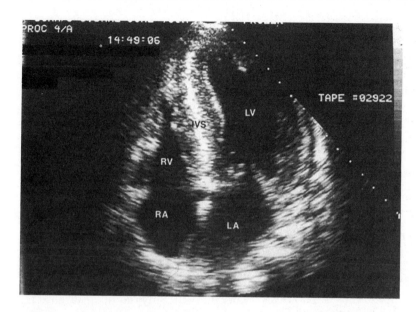

Fig. 8.3 Echocardiogram of a patient with hypertrophic cardiomyopathy. Note the marked asymmetrical hypertrophy of the interventricular septum.

Treatment

Asymptomatic individuals do not require specific drug therapy, although they should probably avoid competitive sporting activities and receive antibiotic prophylaxis against infective endocarditis. Patients with angina or breathlessness may benefit from calcium antagonists such as **verapamil** or **diltiazem**. These improve diastolic filling of the stiff, non-compliant left ventricle by encouraging its relaxation. β-Blockers are

---

Case history

A 24-year-old man presented to his GP because of recurrent faints while playing squash. He was usually extremely fit but had found recently that he was getting more short of breath than usual during his matches. Several times he had blacked out without warning, but on each occasion had recovered quickly. Examination revealed a 'jerky' carotid pulse, a fourth heart sound and an ejection systolic murmur in the aortic area.

Exertional syncope in a young man with these clinical findings is typical of hypertrophic obstructive cardiomyopathy (HOCM). He requires hospital referral to a cardiologist for assessment, including echocardiography and a 24-h ECG. Syncope in HOCM may be due to arrhythmias and may herald sudden death. He should be advised not to exercise until seen by a cardiologist. If the diagnosis is confirmed then he will require genetic counselling and other family members should be screened.

often used and improve ventricular filling mainly by prolonging diastole. Amiodarone is a useful drug if atrial fibrillation or ventricular arrhythmias supervene. Occasionally surgery to resect the thickened interventricular septum or replace an incompetent mitral valve is required. Recent studies also suggest a role for dual chamber pacing in patients with HOCM. Premature apical activation induced by pacing seems to alter favourably the left ventricular contraction pattern. It is important to screen other family members for the condition.

RESTRICTIVE CARDIOMYOPATHY

In this condition the heart is unable to relax effectively, due to a poorly understood process of fibrosis of the endocardium. It behaves rather like constrictive pericarditis, with impaired diastolic filling giving rise to poor cardiac output and high filling pressures. The terminology surrounding this condition is confused. It is often said that restrictive cardiomyopathy is exemplified by amyloidosis. However, with amyloid heart disease the cause, by definition, is known. It is more correct to say that restrictive cardiomyopathy is a condition in which the clinical features closely resemble those associated with amyloid heart disease, but for which no cause can be found. When it occurs in the UK it is often associated with high eosinophil counts, but the condition is more commonly seen in the tropics when it occurs without eosinophilia.

Patients present with oedema and exertional dyspnoea due to high atrial pressures and fluid retention. Examination reveals an elevated JVP with added heart sounds. Routine investigations are often unhelpful with a normal size heart on CXR and non-specific ST–T wave changes

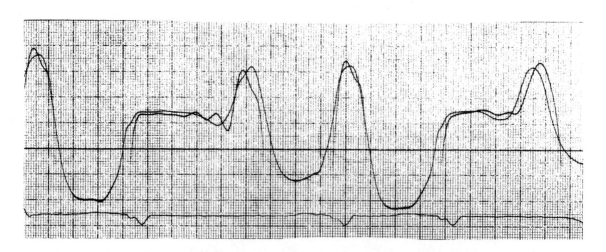

Fig. 8.4 Left ventricular pressure trace of a patient with restrictive cardiomyopathy. The initial diastolic fall is normal but is followed by a plateau as the ventricle will expand no more.

on the ECG. Cardiac catheterization is often needed. This excludes amyloid (by endocardial biopsy) and demonstrates characteristic haemodynamic abnormalities. Relaxation is initially normal, but cardiac distension stops abruptly in mid-diastole. The left ventricular pressure trace shows a normal early diastolic drop, followed by a plateau as the ventricle will expand no more (Fig. 8.4). Fibrosis of the endocardium is often most marked at the ventricular apex and this gives rise to a 'boxing glove' appearance to the left ventricle during contrast angiography.

In addition to conventional heart failure treatment, **resection** of the fibrotic **endocardium** is sometimes beneficial and should be considered.

9 Pericardial disease

The heart is surrounded by the **pericardium**, which fixes the heart in the mediastinum. It consists of three layers. The outermost (**fibrous**) layer blends with the adventitia of the great vessels where they enter and exit the heart. Adherent to the inside of the fibrous pericardium is the **parietal** layer. A small space (the **pericardial space**) separates the parietal layer from the **visceral** layer which covers the heart. The pericardium does not affect myocardial contraction so **systolic function** is well preserved in all forms of pericardial disease. However, abnormalities of the pericardium do have important effects on the ability of the heart to relax and these may dominate the clinical picture in pericardial disease.

PERICARDIAL EFFUSION

Fluid between the parietal and visceral layers of the pericardium is called a **pericardial effusion**. This may be inflammatory fluid, blood or malignant exudate from metastatic deposits in the pericardium. The haemodynamic effects of a pericardial effusion depend partly on its size (volume) but also on its speed of accumulation.

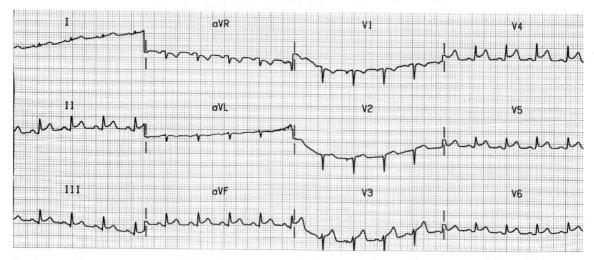

Fig. 9.1 ECG of a patient with a pericardial effusion showing low voltage complexes. There is also S–T elevation in the lateral chest leads. This patient's pericardial effusion was secondary to pericarditis.

Slow accumulation

Symptoms may be absent if accumulation has been gradual as the pericardium is able to stretch gradually and may accommodate a large volume of fluid. Eventually, however, many patients complain of an insidious onset of **breathlessness** and **fatigue**. Clinical signs can be subtle and often the only clue is a quietening of the heart sounds as the presence of extra fluid between the heart and stethoscope attenuates the noises.

Rapid accumulation

Under these circumstances there is no time for the pericardium to stretch and diastolic filling becomes severely inhibited by the presence of fluid in the pericardial space compressing the ventricle from the outside. The heart can only pump out what it has received during diastole so, although contractile function is completely normal, cardiac output is low. In its most severe form this is called **cardiac tamponade**, where impairment of diastolic function causes a severe restriction in cardiac output sufficient to produce tachycardia, hypotension and raised venous pressures with cool clammy peripheries. **Kussmaul's sign** is also frequently seen.

Kussmaul's sign in pericardial effusion

Under normal circumstances inspiration is accompanied by an increase in venous return to the right side of the heart as more blood is 'sucked in' by the fall in intrathoracic pressure. Despite this extra volume of blood pressure in the right side of the heart does not rise. This is because with a greater venous return (preload) the right ventricle is able to increase its output along the Starling curve. With a large, rapidly accumulating pericardial effusion the right ventricle is unable to accommodate this extra volume of blood. Blood remains in the great veins and so, with inspiration, venous pressure rises. A rise in venous pressure with inspiration is called Kussmaul's sign.

Helpful investigations in the diagnosis of pericardial effusion include an ECG (which may show low voltage complexes as the electrical signal is dampened by the presence of extra fluid between the heart and the recording electrodes) (Fig. 9.1) and a CXR which often shows a large, globular shaped heart, usually with clear lung fields (Fig. 9.2). Echocardiography is the investigation of choice and identifies the presence of fluid between the heart and the pericardial sac (Fig. 9.3). It can also show the presence of right ventricular or atrial collapse during diastole which suggests tamponade. However, the urgency with which treatment measures are carried out depends on the patient's haemodynamic condition.

Treatment is by drainage of the accumulated fluid (**pericardiocentesis**). This permits diagnosis (by analysis of the fluid)

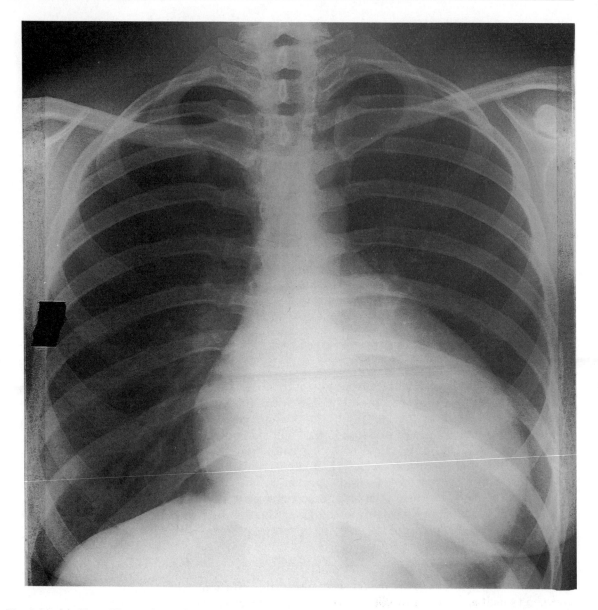

Fig. 9.2 (a) Chest X-ray of a patient with a pericardial effusion, showing a large 'globular' shaped heart and clear lung fields.

and corrects the haemodynamic disturbance. Drainage is usually via a pigtail catheter inserted into the pericardial space under local anaesthetic. This should only be performed by experienced operators with continuous ECG monitoring and full resuscitation equipment at hand.

Pericardial effusions due to metastatic deposits in the pericardium often reaccumulate. One option then is surgical resection of a portion of pericardium. This allows free drainage of the effusion into the

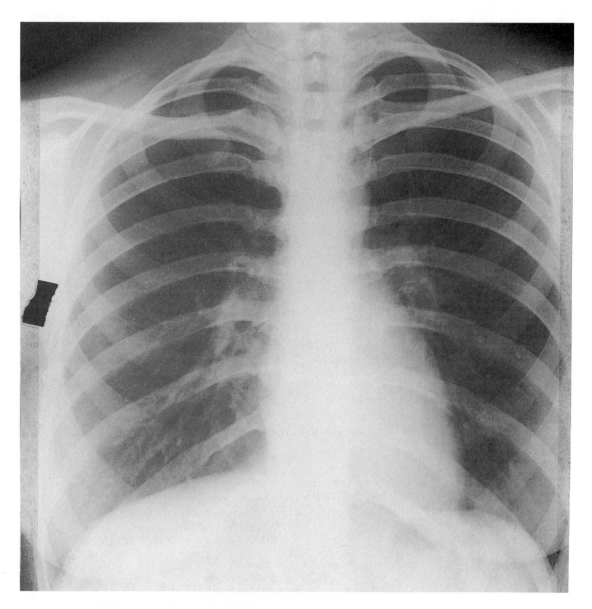

(b) The same patient following pericardiocentesis.

abdominal cavity or mediastinum. The hole created in the pericardium is sometimes called a **pericardial window**.

PERICARDITIS

This is inflammation of the pericardium and can have a number of causes. Most are due to a preceding viral infection, but other causes include connective tissue diseases, post myocardial infarction and renal

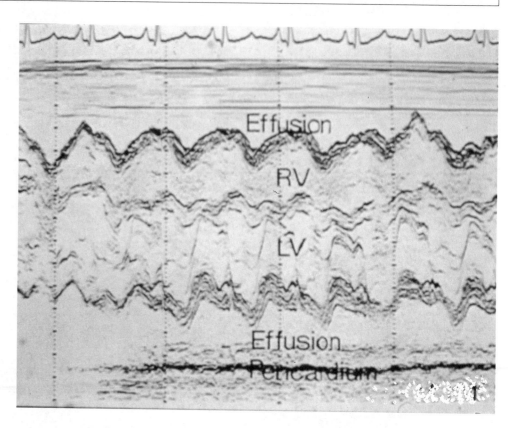

Fig. 9.3 M mode echocardiogram of a patient with a pericardial effusion.

Causes of pericardial effusion	
Blood	Following cardiac surgery Myocardial infarction with rupture of ventricular wall Aortic dissection/aneurysm with rupture into the pericardium
Malignant exudate	Breast and lung are the commonest deposits
Inflammatory fluid	Viral/bacterial/tuberculous pericarditis Renal failure

failure. Tuberculous pericarditis is now uncommon. The layers of the pericardium become inflamed, so when they move over one another during systole and diastole they cause an intense stabbing central chest pain which is classically relieved by sitting forward and worsened by deep respiration. Symptoms of cardiac failure are rare unless there is an accompanying pericardial effusion.

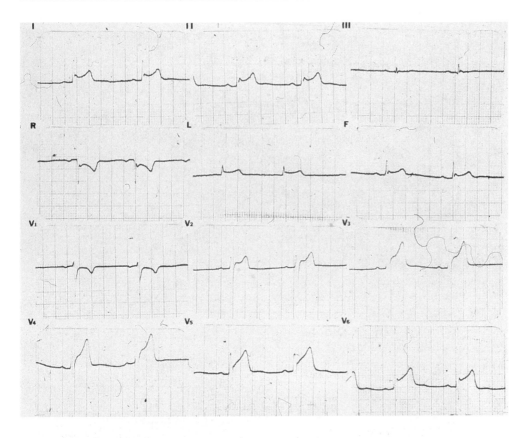

Fig. 9.4 ECG of a patient with acute pericarditis. Note the widespread concave upwards S–T segment elevation.

Case history

A 39-year-old woman with known ovarian cancer presented to Casualty with rapidly increasing breathlessness. She had been well until two days previously when she became unusually breathless running for a bus. Things worsened steadily and by the time of her arrival she was very short of breath at rest. On examination she was cold, clammy and unwell with a fast, weak pulse. The Casualty doctor found it difficult to take her blood pressure as the Korotkoff sounds seemed to be variable in their intensity. Heart sounds were almost inaudible. A 12-lead ECG showed very small complexes and a CXR revealed a huge globular shaped heart.

These are the typical features of a pericardial effusion. This patient requires urgent echocardiography to confirm the diagnosis and removal of the fluid (pericardiocentesis). In this case the likeliest cause of the effusion is pericardial metastases from the ovarian cancer.

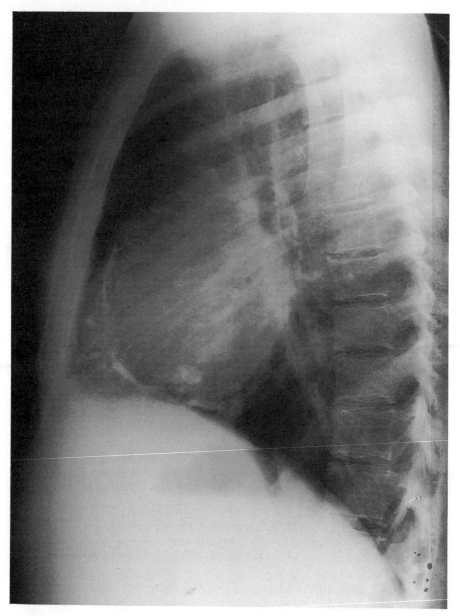

Fig. 9.5 Lateral chest X-ray of a patient with calcific tuberculous pericarditis.

Examination often reveals a **pericardial friction rub**. This is a scratchy noise best appreciated at the left sternal edge with the diaphragm of the stethoscope. It may be heard at any point in the cardiac cycle and seems to the listener to be very close to the chest wall.

Investigations may be normal in pericarditis. Most helpful is the ECG which classically shows S–T segment elevation in several leads, with the

concave shape pointing **upwards** (Fig. 9.4). The CXR usually shows no abnormality unless there is a pericardial effusion, which can be detected by echocardiography.

Treatment is largely symptomatic, with NSAIDs being the most helpful drugs. A pericardial friction rub in the context of renal failure is an indication for dialysis.

CONSTRICTIVE PERICARDITIS

Virtually any cause of acute pericarditis may go on to cause diffuse fibrosis of the pericardium. It classically follows radiation to the chest or tuberculous pericarditis, although the latter is now rare. Again, diastolic function is impaired as the heart effectively becomes encased in a rigid shell. End-diastolic pressures in both ventricles are high as venous return flows into chambers that are unable to expand and accommodate the blood.

Left- and right-sided cardiac output is limited causing symptoms of fatigue and weight loss (poor left-sided output) and peripheral oedema with ascites (low right-sided output). There may be a history of previous pericarditis, tuberculosis, cardiac surgery or radiation treatment.

Examination reveals a low volume pulse, oedema, ascites and high venous pressures. The diagnostic value of classically quoted signs such as pulsus paradoxus and a rapid y descent to the JVP are perhaps overstated and do not merit discussion here. Sometimes a diastolic sound called a **pericardial knock** is heard. This is actually a very loud third heart sound produced when rapid ventricular filling is abruptly halted as the rigid pericardium will expand no more.

Routine investigations are often unhelpful. The ECG may show non-specific T wave changes but the classical pericardial calcification seen on lateral CXR of patients with tuberculous pericarditis is now rare (Fig. 9.5). Cardiac catheterization is needed to confirm the diagnosis which shows raised and equal end diastolic pressures in the ventricles and atria.

Treatment is by surgical removal of the pericardium (**pericardiectomy**).

10 | Congenital heart disease

EMBRYOLOGICAL BACKGROUND

During fetal life, blood is oxygenated by the placenta rather than the lungs. The lungs are not aerated and there is little flow through the pulmonary circulation. Blood therefore 'bypasses' the lungs and is diverted into the systemic circulation, where demand for oxygen in the developing tissues (particularly the brain) is high. This is achieved by a combination of two connecting vessels (**ducts**) and a valve system between the two atria; all of which close shortly after birth to create the adult circulation. A schematic diagram of the fetal circulation is shown below (Fig. 10.1).

Oxygenated blood from the umbilical veins passes through the **ductus venosus** into the inferior vena cava. From here it enters the right atrium but is then diverted into the left atrium by the valve-like action of the **fossa ovalis**. Once in the left atrium blood exits the heart as in the adult, via the left ventricle and aorta. Venous return to the heart from

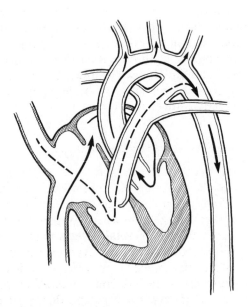

Fig. 10.1 Schematic diagram of the fetal circulation.

the head and neck is via the superior vena cava. It forms a **separate stream** in the right atrium and is directed into the right ventricle. From here blood passes into the pulmonary trunk, but very high resistances in the pulmonary circulation discourage further flow. The **ductus arteriosus** connects the pulmonary trunk to the descending aorta, so the pulmonary circulation is 'bypassed'. Patency of the ductus arteriosus is maintained by prostaglandin synthesis within its wall. Blood in the descending aorta then returns to the placenta via the umbilical artery for oxygenation.

CHANGES WITH BIRTH

At birth the baby takes a breath for the first time. Aeration of lung tissue reduces pulmonary resistance. This promotes pulmonary blood flow, which in turn increases flow and pressure in the left atrium. This closes the valve that previously allowed blood to flow from right to left atrium and this communication is lost.

A combination of factors causes the ductus arteriosus to close. Pulmonary resistance falls with aeration of lung tissue so the pressure in the pulmonary trunk that previously favoured flow down the duct also falls. In addition rising levels of oxygen and falling levels of prostaglandins cause **vasoconstriction** of the duct, which reduces flow further. The lungs are no longer bypassed and the adult arrangement of pulmonary and systemic circulations in series is established. Clamping of the placenta at birth abolishes flow in the ductus venosus. This duct also responds to increased oxygen and decreased prostaglandin levels by constricting, leaving a cord-like remnant.

Congenital heart disease may result when these changes fail to occur or if the initial development of the structures involved is 'faulty'. In most cases of congenital heart disease the cause is unknown, but a few are associated with chromosomal abnormalities such as Down's syndrome (a third of Down's babies have structural heart defects), or with maternal viral infections (such as rubella) during the first trimester of pregnancy.

Cyanotic and acyanotic congenital heart disease

The changes that occur around the time of birth ensure that deoxygenated blood flows through the pulmonary circulation, where it picks up oxygen. From here it returns to the left side of the heart and is directed into the systemic circulation where oxygen is released and taken up by metabolizing tissues. Congenital defects may be divided on the basis of whether they produce **cyanosis**. Cyanosis refers to the purplish coloration seen in mucous membranes when a sufficient quantity of deoxygenated blood enters the systemic circulation. Any congenital lesion in which a significant quantity of deoxygenated blood is misdirected ('shunted') from the right to the left side of the heart (thereby 'bypassing' the opportunity to be oxygenated) will produce cyanosis. These are called 'right to left shunts' and cyanosis, with its important effects on growth and development, dominates the clinical picture. Defects that cause blood to flow from the left to the right heart will not cause cyanosis because the blood is merely doing an 'extra circuit' of the lungs. These are called 'left to right shunts' and their main effect is to increase the amount of blood flowing through the pulmonary circulation.

Eisenmenger syndrome

Sometimes patients with congenital defects that start as 'left to right shunts' go on to develop cyanosis at a later stage. This is because the increased volume of blood flowing through the lungs causes changes in the pulmonary vasculature with chronic vasoconstriction. This increases resistance to blood flow through the lungs, causing **pulmonary hypertension**. Eventually pressure in the right ventricle exceeds that in the left ventricle, blood flows from right to left and the shunt is said to have **reversed**. A left to right shunt which subsequently reverses due to pulmonary hypertension is called the **Eisenmenger syndrome**. The initial abnormality may be a hole in the atrium (**atrial septal defect**), a hole in the ventricle (**ventricular septal defect**) or a ductus arteriosus that has failed to close (**patent ductus arteriosus**).

ACYANOTIC CONGENITAL HEART LESIONS

Atrial septal defect

In this condition there is an abnormal connection between the two atria across the atrial septum. Pressures in the left atrium are higher than the right, so blood flows across the septum producing a left to right shunt. There are several anatomical variants of atrial septal defect (ASD) that relate to defects in the developing structures of the heart. It is not necessary to know the detailed embryology except that defects lower down the septum (called **primum** defects) may also involve the mitral valve and cause mitral regurgitation. The commoner (**secundum**) type is not associated with mitral regurgitation (Fig. 10.2).

Clinical features

Left to right atrial communication means that some oxygenated blood returning from the lungs does an 'extra loop' of the pulmonary circulation. The clinical effects of this depend on the size of the defect and therefore the amount of flow across the shunt. **Small shunts** are often asymptomatic until middle age when they are detected during routine examination or may present with atrial arrhythmias (particularly atrial fibrillation). Some patients develop symptoms and signs of heart failure. Right heart failure develops because of the effect

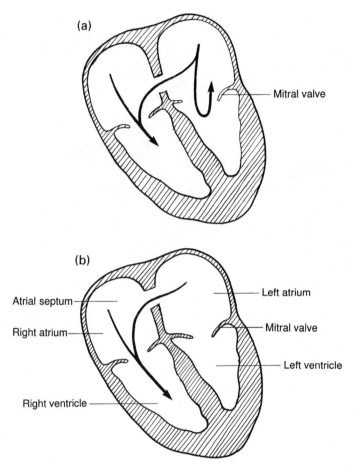

(a)

Mitral valve

(b)

Atrial septum

Right atrium

Right ventricle

Left atrium

Mitral valve

Left ventricle

Fig. 10.2 Atrial septal defects. (a) Primum and (b) secundum defects.

of chronic volume loading on the right ventricle. Breathlessness and fatigue occur because systemic cardiac output is not adequate for exercise as blood is misdirected back into the right side of the heart instead of into the left ventricle and aorta. With **large shunts** symptoms and signs usually develop in childhood. Children may suffer repeated respiratory infections, develop exertional dyspnoea or simply 'fail to thrive'. Occasionally large shunts, if left untreated for a long time, progress to an **Eisenmenger syndrome** as described above.

The auscultatory findings are similar for all types of ASD. The right ventricle takes longer to complete its emptying due to the extra volume of blood that it has acquired from flow across the atrial septum. Consequently, closure of the pulmonary valve (P_2) is delayed and becomes more distinct from A_2. Blood continues to flow across the atrial septum irrespective of the phase of the respiratory cycle (recall that venous return to the right ventricle increases during inspiration). There is no effect on the timing of P_2 with respiration and the second heart

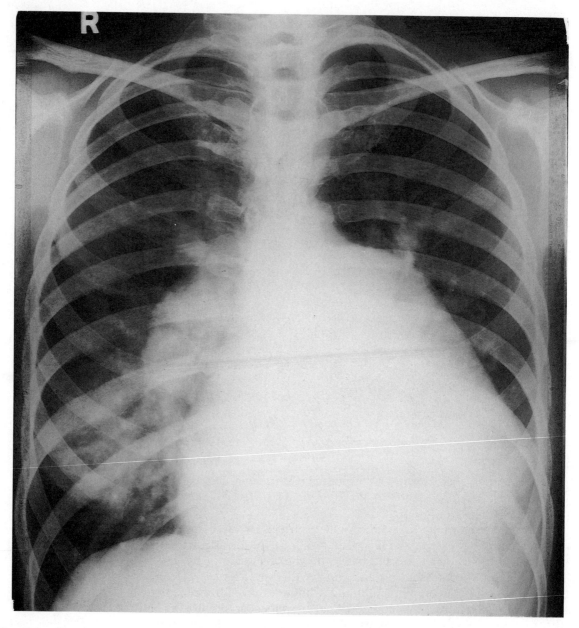

Fig. 10.3 Chest X-ray of a patient with ASD showing cardiomegaly, large pulmonary arteries and pulmonary plethora.

sound is therefore said to be **fixed and widely split**. The extra volume of blood flowing across the pulmonary valve may cause an ejection systolic murmur in that area. The murmur of mitral regurgitation may be heard with primum defects. The presence of cyanosis and signs of heart failure depend on the size and duration of the shunt as discussed above.

Investigations

The CXR in ASD shows a large heart with prominent pulmonary arteries and plethoric lung fields due to the increased flow through the lungs (Fig. 10.3). The ECG typically shows right bundle branch block, sometimes with right ventricular hypertrophy. There is often left axis deviation with primum defects. Echocardiography usually identifies enlarged right-sided chambers but demonstrating the abnormal flow across the atrial septum can be difficult on Doppler studies. Cardiac catheterization is the definitive investigation. Blood samples from the right atrium are more oxygenated than blood in the superior and inferior vena cavae, indicating that there has been some mixing with blood from the left atrium. This is called a **step-up** in saturation. It is possible to calculate how much more blood is flowing through the lungs than the systemic circulation from the amount of step-up in saturation.

Treatment

This depends on the size of the shunt. If pulmonary blood flow is more than 1.5 times systemic flow then surgical closure is usually advised, even in the absence of symptoms, as most such patients develop cardiac failure or, troublesome arrhythmias in middle age. Symptomatic ASDs in infancy require early closure to allow normal growth and development. ASDs complicated by Eisenmenger syndrome can only be treated with **heart–lung transplantation** as the right ventricle of a simple heart transplant would quickly fail against the high pulmonary pressures. Antibiotic prophylaxis is advised for all patients with ASD.

Case history

A 28-year-old man underwent cardiac catheterization as part of the investigation of a heart murmur. The following values were recorded.

	Pressure (mmHg)	Saturation (%)
SVC	–	62
IVC	–	65
RA	5	85
RV	45/5	88
PA	45/15	89
Ao	100/70	97

These are typical findings in an ASD. There is a step-up in saturation in the RA, indicating that this chamber has acquired oxygenated blood. The pressures in the right ventricle and pulmonary artery are increased as a consequence of the increased flow through the pulmonary circulation. Operation to close the ASD was advised.

Ventricular septal defect

In this condition a hole in the interventricular septum allows movement of blood between the two ventricles (Fig. 10.4). In the first few days of life there is little flow across the defect as pulmonary and right heart pressures are still falling from their high intrauterine levels. Right ventricular pressure then falls gradually so that by a month a left to right shunt is established, as blood is forced across the septum by the higher pressures in the left ventricle. Again, symptoms and signs depend largely on the size of the defect and therefore the volume of blood flowing through the shunt.

Clinical features

Small shunts do not usually cause symptoms. The effect of a high pressure in the left ventricle driving blood through a small hole creates a very loud murmur, so most small VSDs are detected on routine examination. Larger defects allow a greater flow of blood across the septum so pulmonary blood flow is increased at the expense of systemic cardiac output. Presentation is usually in childhood with breathlessness, fatigue or failure to thrive. Eisenmenger's syndrome may complicate large shunts.

Examination of patients with small shunts may be normal except for the characteristic murmur. This is **pansystolic** as pressure in the left ventricle exceeds that in the right ventricle for virtually the whole cardiac cycle. With larger defects a variable amount of right and left ventricular hypertrophy may be detected. The RV hypertrophies in response to the large volume of blood in that chamber. The LV hypertrophies in an attempt to generate an adequate systemic cardiac output. Consequently, a parasternal heave and/or displaced apex beat may be felt. Larger VSDs are generally associated with softer murmurs

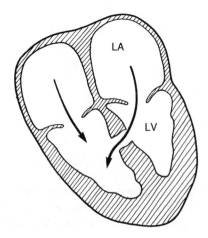

Fig. 10.4 Ventricular septal defect.

as there is less obstruction to blood flow between the two ventricles. Cyanosis is apparent in Eisenmenger's syndrome.

Investigations

These may be normal with a small defect. With larger defects the ECG shows left and/or right ventricular hypertrophy. CXR shows biventricular enlargement with prominent pulmonary arteries and plethoric lung fields due to the large flow of blood through the lungs. Echocardiography may identify the abnormal jet of blood, although the anatomical defect may be difficult to visualize. Cardiac catheterization includes a study of both sides of the heart. When the right heart is catheterized a step up in oxygenation is seen in the right ventricle, analogous to that seen in ASD. During a left ventricular angiogram a jet of dye can be seen passing through the defect into the right ventricle.

Treatment

Small VSDs require no treatment and many close spontaneously with time. Larger defects should be closed surgically in order to protect the pulmonary circulation and prevent Eisenmenger's syndrome. All patients with VSD should receive prophylactic antibiotics as the risk of endocarditis is high.

Patent ductus arteriosus

Strictly speaking this should be called a persistent patent ductus arteriosus (PDA) as all people have a patent ductus *in utero*. If the ductus fails to close after birth then a communication is left between the

---

Case history

An 18-year-old man underwent cardiac catheterization as part of the investigation of a heart murmur present since childhood. The following values were obtained.

	Pressure (mmHg)	Oxygen saturation (%)
SVC	–	68
IVC	–	72
RA	4	68
RV	37/9	82
PA	38/10	83
LV	105/0	97

These are the classical findings of a VSD. There is a step-up in saturation from the RA to the RV. In other words the RV has acquired oxygenated blood from the LV across a VSD to increase the saturation level.

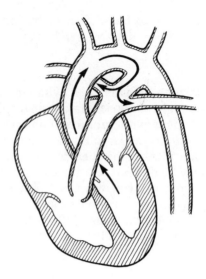

Fig. 10.5 Patent ductus arteriosus.

descending aorta (beyond the origin of the head and neck vessels) and the pulmonary trunk (Fig. 10.5). Even with a patent duct blood flow down this vessel immediately after birth is minimal as pressures in the pulmonary circulation are still relatively high. Within a few weeks pulmonary artery pressure has fallen to adult levels and a gradient is established across the duct, with high pressures in the aorta driving blood through the duct into the lower pressure pulmonary system. Pulmonary blood flow is therefore high at the expense of systemic output.

Examination

Typically there is a collapsing pulse. Blood ejected into the aorta during systole rapidly runs off into the pulmonary circulation through the duct, so diastolic pressure is reduced. The left ventricle attempts to compensate for this by increasing the force of contraction, causing the characteristic rapid upstroke of the collapsing pulse. The haemodynamic effects on the left ventricle are similar to those of aortic regurgitation. Blood that flows down the duct does an extra circuit of the lungs and is added to normal pulmonary venous return in the next cardiac cycle. This chronically **volume loads** the left ventricle and with time patients may develop heart failure. Aortic pressure exceeds pulmonary artery pressure for the whole of the cardiac cycle so the murmur of a PDA is continuous and often described as 'machinery like'. It is best heard in the left second interspace. As with other left to right shunts Eisenmenger syndrome may develop and patients with PDA are at significant risk of endocarditis.

Investigations

These may include prominent pulmonary arteries on CXR (due to the extra volume of blood flowing through the lungs) and left ventricular hypertrophy on the ECG as this chamber attempts to maintain systemic cardiac output. Echocardiography shows dilated left-sided chambers and Doppler studies identify abnormal blood flow within the duct. Right heart catheterization demonstrates a step up in oxygen saturation in the pulmonary trunk where oxygenated aortic blood joins deoxygenated blood from the right ventricle.

Treatment

The ducts of premature infants may close with indomethacin, which inhibits the synthesis of the prostaglandins that help maintain duct patency *in utero*. Where this fails, all PDAs require treatment with **surgical ligation** or percutaneous placement of an umbrella-like device that occludes the PDA. Morbidity associated with either procedure is low and the risk of endocarditis is almost abolished.

Coarctation of the aorta

In this condition there is a localized narrowing of the aorta, usually beyond the origin of the head and neck vessels (Fig. 10.6). It may be caused by the presence of tissue from the ductus arteriosus in the wall of the aorta. Hence, when the ductus constricts after birth a similar process occurs in the aorta causing the narrowing. Important associations with coarctation include Berry aneurysms in the cerebral circulation and a

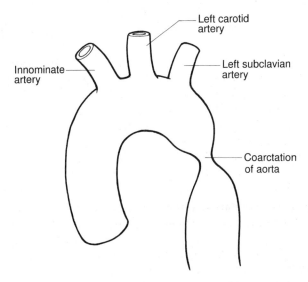

Fig. 10.6   Coarctation of the aorta.

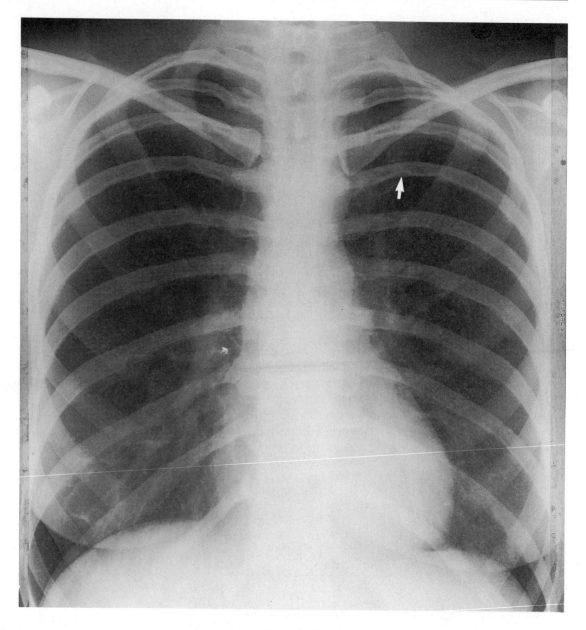

Fig. 10.7 Chest X-ray of a patient with coarctation. Rib notching can clearly be seen (arrowed).

bicuspid aortic valve. Patients may present with complications of these such as subarachnoid haemorrhage or aortic stenosis.

Clinical features

Severe coarctation presents early in life with heart failure as the left ventricle is unable to cope with the strain of maintaining output across the tight narrowing. A more usual presentation is later in life with hypertension. The left ventricle undergoes hypertrophy in order to try and maintain flow across the obstructed aorta. A combination of this and high renin levels (from reduced renal perfusion) produces hypertension in the upper limbs, with lower blood pressure in the legs. It is important to exclude coarctation in all young hypertensive patients. The fibrous narrowing in the aorta retards transmission of the pulse wave to the legs, so the femoral pulses occur well after the radial pulses from the same ventricular contraction. This is called **radio-femoral delay**. Turbulent flow through the narrowed segment may produce a systolic murmur. Bruits may be heard from the collateral circulation described below.

Investigations

The CXR in coarctation is characteristic. Faced with an obstruction just beyond the aortic arch blood reaches the distal aorta through an extensive collateral circulation, mainly involving the intercostal vessels. These become dilated due to the increased flow of blood and may erode into the underside of the ribs (typically numbers 4–8). Thus, **rib-notching** is the classical radiological sign of coarctation (Fig. 10.7). The ECG shows left ventricular hypertrophy. Although coarctation may be seen with echocardiography, cardiac catheterization may be needed to define its extent. In recent years the use of MRI scanning to define the anatomy of coarctation has become more widespread (Fig. 10.8).

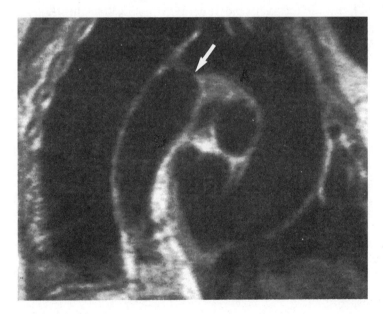

Fig. 10.8   MRI scan of a patient with coarctation of the aorta. The narrowing can clearly be seen (arrowed).

Treatment

This is generally by surgical resection of the narrowed segment. If it is too long to allow end to end anastomosis a graft may be required. Surgical resection does not always correct hypertension. There is a 10% incidence of recoarctation following surgical resection, when balloon dilatation is the treatment of choice.

CYANOTIC CONGENITAL HEART DISEASE

Fallot's tetralogy

Although, by definition, this condition has four components the haemodynamic disturbance can be understood by considering just two: a **ventricular septal defect** and **subpulmonary stenosis**. The obstruction to flow out of the right ventricle means that deoxygenated blood is 'shunted' across the VSD into the left ventricle, bypassing the lungs and causing cyanosis (Fig. 10.9). The 'tighter' the subpulmonary stenosis the greater the head of pressure forcing blood from right to left away from the lungs and the more severe the cyanosis. The other two components of the tetralogy are **right ventricular hypertrophy** (which occurs in response to the obstruction to pulmonary blood flow) and an aorta which 'overrides' the VSD. This is an anatomical abnormality that means the mouth of the aorta lies over the VSD as well as being the outlet of the left ventricle. Consequently, deoxygenated blood from the right ventricle can flow directly into the aorta without first passing through the VSD into the left ventricle. It actually makes little difference to the degree of cyanosis but does make the anatomy more difficult for the surgeon.

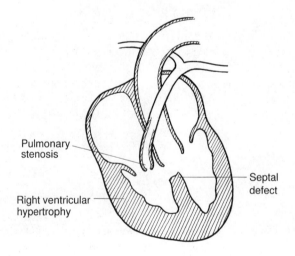

Pulmonary stenosis

Septal defect

Right ventricular hypertrophy

Fig. 10.9 Tetralogy of Fallot.

Clinical features

If the subpulmonary stenosis is severe then presentation is in infancy with cyanosis, episodes of apnoea, breathlessness and failure to thrive. With moderate degrees of stenosis more blood can 'get past' the obstruction into the pulmonary circulation for oxygenation. Presentation therefore tends to be later with **episodic cyanosis**. The obstruction to outflow from the right ventricle is due to thickened muscle below the pulmonary valve rather than an abnormality of the valve itself. If this muscle 'tightens up' then outflow is further impeded and a greater head of pressure in the right ventricle drives blood across the VSD into the systemic circulation. Children often squat on their haunches to relieve symptoms of breathlessness. This manoeuvre increases systemic resistance so that shunting of blood into the aorta is less favoured and more blood is driven into the pulmonary circulation. With very mild degrees of stenosis sufficient blood may get into the pulmonary circulation to prevent cyanosis altogether. This is called **acyanotic Fallot's** and presentation is as for a simple VSD.

Examination

This may reveal **cyanosis**, **clubbing** and poor physical development. There may be an **ejection systolic murmur** generated by flow through the narrowed right ventricular outflow tract. P_2 is usually absent as insufficient blood gets into the pulmonary circulation to close the valve with the necessary force to generate a sound. It is this that distinguishes Fallot's from an Eisenmenger's VSD, where pulmonary hypertension closes the pulmonary valve with increased force, generating a loud P_2.

Investigations

The CXR in Fallot's shows marked right ventricular enlargement which lifts the apex away from the diaphragm 'towards 3 o'clock'. In addition there is so little blood getting past the pulmonary valve that the pulmonary arteries are very small. The combination of a lack of pulmonary artery shadow on the left and the elevated apex gives the heart the characteristic 'boot shape' (Fig. 10.10). The ECG shows right ventricular hypertrophy. Echocardiography identifies the VSD, the overriding aorta and the abnormal flow patterns on Doppler. Cardiac catheterization is essential to quantitate the degree of subpulmonary stenosis.

Treatment

If the stenosis is very severe, causing a large right to left shunt, then a palliative procedure is required to buy time and allow normal growth and development prior to definitive treatment. This is achieved with a **Blalock–Taussig shunt**, which redirects blood from the subclavian artery

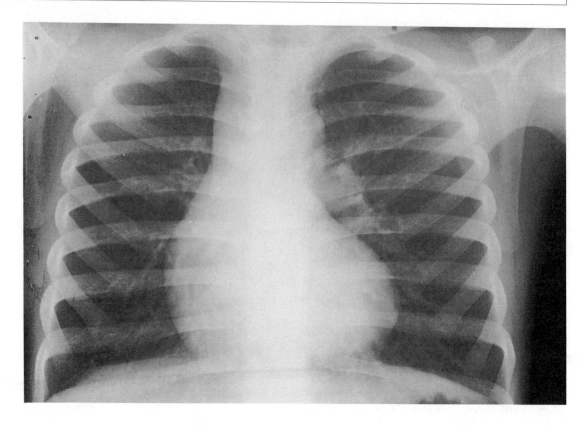

Fig. 10.10   Chest X-ray of a patient with Tetralogy of Fallot, showing oligaemic lung fields, small pulmonary arteries and a 'boot-shaped' heart.

into the pulmonary trunk for oxygenation. Correction of the pulmonary stenosis and closure of the VSD is carried out at a later date. An increasing number of patients have undergone total correction without a prior shunt.

Transposition of the great arteries

This condition may be thought of as a 'plumbing problem' in which the ventricles are connected to the wrong outflow vessel. The right ventricle pumps blood into the aorta and the left ventricle is connected to the pulmonary trunk. This produces severe cyanosis immediately after birth. Babies are dependent on blood from the two sides mixing and this is usually through an associated ASD. If there is no connection then babies quickly become critically ill and the immediate management is to create an ASD by dragging a percutaneously inserted balloon through the atrial septum (balloon septostomy). Definitive surgical treatment involves removing the atrial septum and redirecting the two streams of blood into the correct ventricle (the Senning procedure). However, this leaves the thinner walled right ventricle responsible for maintaining the

Case history

A child of 12 months underwent cardiac catheterization as part of the investigation for recurrent cyanotic attacks. The following values were recorded.

	Pressure (mmHg)	Saturation (%)
SVC	–	66
IVC	–	70
RA	3	70
RV	98/7	69
PA	16/6	68
LA	9	96
LV	100/0	85
Aorta	100/65	82

These are the features of Fallot's tetralogy. There is a large gradient across the pulmonary valve. Oxygenated blood returns from the lungs through the LA but there is a significant step-down in saturation in the LV, indicating that this chamber has acquired deoxygenated blood from the RV across a VSD.

systemic circulation and, with time, it may fail. A newer procedure is the arterial switch operation which, although technically difficult, aims to correct the anatomical problems.

Pulmonary stenosis

Obstruction to the outlet of the right ventricle may be due to fusion of the leaflets of the pulmonary valve or because the muscle underneath the valve 'grows into' the outflow tract (subvalvular or subpulmonary stenosis). The effect is the same, with a reduced amount of blood getting into the pulmonary circulation for oxygenation. Mild cases are asymptomatic, but if the obstruction is more severe then patients present with breathlessness or exertional syncope as the right ventricle cannot increase its delivery of blood for oxygenation during exercise. The right ventricle becomes 'pressure loaded' against the high resistance to outflow and, with time, may fail.

Examination

This reveals a **parasternal heave** from the overworked right ventricle and an **ejection systolic murmur** in the pulmonary area due to turbulent flow across the narrowed valve. The right ventricle takes longer to complete its emptying due to the obstruction, so P_2 is delayed. If the stenosis is very severe then there may be insufficient blood in the pulmonary circulation to generate a heart sound and P_2 may be absent.

Investigations

These show right ventricular hypertrophy on ECG and a paucity of blood in the lung fields on CXR. Paradoxically the pulmonary arteries may be large, due to **post-stenotic dilatation**. Doppler studies can quantify the gradient across the valve.

Treatment

Treatment of pulmonary valve stenosis is usually by dilating the valve orifice with a balloon inserted percutaneously and passed through the right ventricle. The prognosis is excellent. Subvalvular stenosis requires surgical intervention.

Complex congenital heart disease

This chapter has described some of the more common congenital lesions. It is important to appreciate, however, that many patients present with combinations of these and other, more rare, cardiac defects. It is often impossible, even for experienced doctors, to make the diagnosis clinically and frequently the complexity of the problem is apparent only after echocardiography or cardiac catheterization.

Miscellaneous conditions

ATRIAL MYXOMA

Myxomas are benign cardiac tumours that may arise from anywhere within the heart lining, but usually from the interatrial septum. Most extend into the left atrium where, if sufficiently large, they may obstruct the mitral valve. A common presentation of left atrial myxoma is therefore with orthopnoea, exertional dyspnoea and auscultatory findings similar to mitral stenosis. Obstruction of the mitral valve is intermittent so the clinical findings may be variable. Sometimes a characteristic diastolic sound is heard (a 'plop') as the tumour falls through the mitral valve and hits the left ventricle. Other important presentations include stroke or transient ischaemic episodes from recurrent embolism of tumour; and a systemic illness resembling lupus or infective endocarditis due to an immunological reaction against the

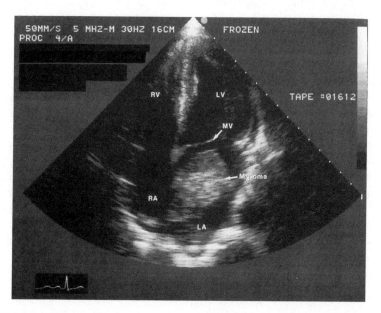

Fig. 11.1   Echocardiogram of a left atrial myxoma showing a mass in the left atrium.

tumour. By analogy right atrial myxomas may present with right heart failure, due to tricuspid valve obstruction, or with pulmonary embolism.

Echocardiography demonstrates the tumour clearly (Fig. 11.1). The ESR is usually raised and patients are often anaemic. Treatment is with urgent surgical excision.

PULMONARY EMBOLISM

Embolism refers to the process whereby a vessel becomes occluded by something that originated at a distant site. The occluding matter is most commonly blood clot but other, more rare, causes of embolism include air, fat and tumour. Occlusion of pulmonary arteries in this way is called pulmonary embolism (PE). It most commonly occurs when a piece of clot breaks off from a more extensive area of thrombosis in a pelvic or leg vein and passes through the right side of the heart to lodge in a pulmonary artery or arteries. PE may present either as an acute event or as a more insidious process in which multiple (usually clinically silent) episodes of embolism gradually occlude more and more of the pulmonary circulation.

Acute pulmonary embolism

Sudden occlusion of a sufficient portion of the pulmonary vascular tree by clot causes sudden onset of breathlessness. If blood cannot get to a significant number of alveoli because of clot in the pulmonary arteries then regardless of how well those alveoli are ventilated there will be submaximal oxygenation of blood, which causes breathlessness. The substance of the lung (the parenchyma) can usually survive on blood delivered by the bronchial arteries which arise from the thoracic aorta and are therefore unaffected by pulmonary embolism. However, if this circulation is not adequate then a portion of lung may die and **pulmonary infarction** is said to have occurred. This may cause **pleuritic chest pain** and/or **haemoptysis**. These symptoms do not occur in pulmonary embolism unless there has been infarction.

Occlusion of more than 50% of the pulmonary arteries is described as **massive pulmonary embolism** and in addition to breathlessness causes dramatic haemodynamic disturbance. The right ventricle is unable to drive enough blood through the lungs into the left heart due to the obstructing clot. The left ventricle can only pump out the blood it has acquired from pulmonary venous return, so despite completely normal contraction cardiac output is limited. In its most severe form this can cause shock with tachycardia, hypotension and oliguria.

Examination

Examination may show evidence of deep venous thrombosis. If this is not evident, rectal and/or vaginal examinations may be appropriate to look

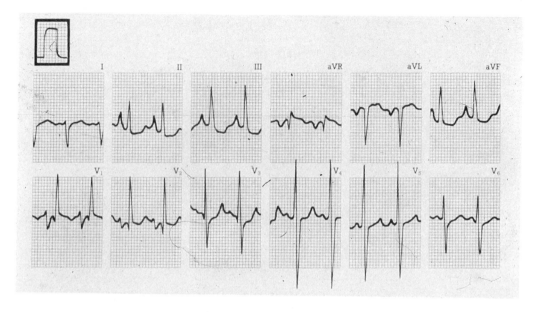

Fig. 11.2 Acute right heart strain shown on the ECG of a patient with pulmonary embolism. Note the QRS complexes are all positive in lead III and negative in lead I, indicating right axis deviation. The P waves in the inferior leads are tall and 'peaked' indicating right atrial strain.

for evidence of pelvic malignancy. Patients with sizeable emboli are usually **tachypnoeic** and **tachycardic**. Sudden onset of atrial fibrillation is a well recognized association. **Venous pressure** may be **raised** as the right ventricular outflow is obstructed by the partially occluded pulmonary circulation. A **pleural rub** is heard in some patients with pulmonary infarction. Massive pulmonary embolism causes sympathetic activation with sweaty, clammy peripheries and hypotension.

Routine investigations are often abnormal only in large PEs. Arterial blood gases show **hypoxia** if a significant portion of lung is unavailable for gas transfer; and **hypocapnia** from the reactive overbreathing secondary to this. The ECG in PE classically shows one or all of the following: a deep S wave in lead I and a Q wave with an inverted T wave in lead III. S–T depression with T inversion in the right ventricular leads (V_1 and V_2) indicate severe acute right heart strain from the obstruction to pulmonary blood flow (Fig. 11.2). CXR may show a pleural effusion. Occasionally, if there has been pulmonary infarction, a wedge-shaped radiolucent area next to the pleurae may be seen. Necrosis of a pulmonary infarct may cause a cavitating lesion on CXR.

Investigations

Special investigations are usually required to make the diagnosis. The **ventilation/perfusion (V/P) scan** (Fig. 11.3) is most often used and relies

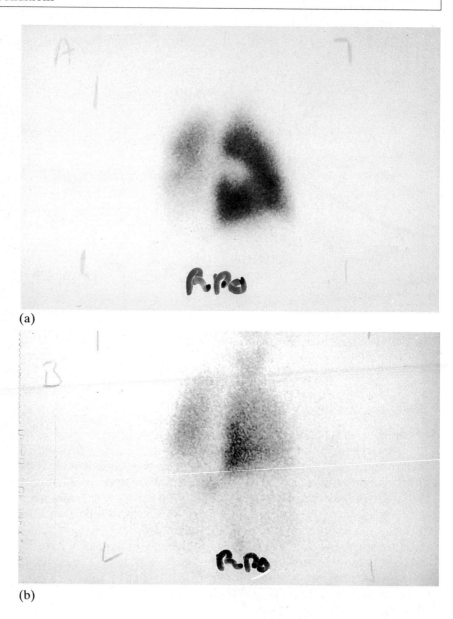

(a)

(b)

Fig. 11.3 Ventilation perfusion scan in pulmonary embolism. There is a defect in the apical segment of the right lower lobe on the perfusion scan (a) which is not present on the ventilation scan (b). This is typical of pulmonary embolism.

on the principle that ventilation of an area of lung affected by pulmonary embolus is normal whereas perfusion, by definition, is not.

Pulmonary angiography is the gold standard for the diagnosis of pulmonary embolism but is only carried out in cases of massive PE if surgical intervention is being considered (Fig. 11.4).

Minor PEs are treated with oxygen and subcutaneous heparin, followed by anticoagulation with warfarin for 3–6 months. Massive

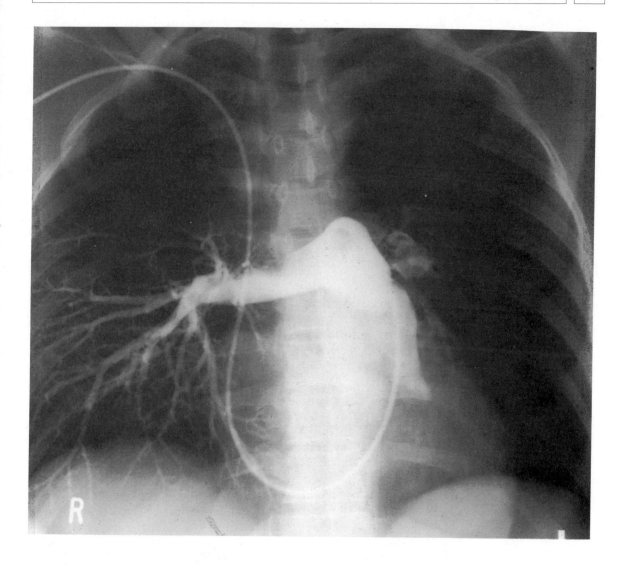

Fig. 11.4 Pulmonary angiogram in massive pulmonary embolism, showing absence of dye in the right upper lobe and throughout the left lung.

pulmonary embolism requires oxygen and heparin, but also intravenous fluids and inotropic support where necessary. Streptokinase may be given to lyse the clot and in extreme cases embolectomy may be required.

Chronic pulmonary embolism

Sometimes several 'mini-clots' lodge in the pulmonary circulation, which causes an insidious increase in the obstruction to blood flow through the lungs. In such cases the source of clots and their embolism

Ventilation/perfusion scans

In this investigation the blood pool is made temporarily radioactive by an injection of ^{99}technetium. Areas of lung where the supplying pulmonary artery has been occluded by thrombus will show as **perfusion defects** when the lungs are scanned with a gamma counter. Perfusion defects are non-specific and may also be caused by pneumonia or chronic bronchitis. The patient then breathes in air made temporarily radioactive with an isotope of xenon. In pulmonary embolism there is nothing wrong with the alveoli, so the ventilation scan recorded by the gamma counter shows no defects. If an area of lung is ventilated but not perfused a **ventilation/perfusion mismatch** is said to exist and this is highly suggestive of pulmonary embolism.

is often clinically silent. Up to a point the right ventricle is able to compensate by hypertrophy, but eventually it is unable to maintain satisfactory pulmonary blood flow and patients develop exertional breathlessness. Examination reveals raised venous pressures, oedema and a loud P_2 as the high pulmonary pressures close the pulmonary valve forcefully. Treatment is with lifelong anticoagulation.

Case history
A 32-year-old woman was brought to hospital by ambulance acutely breathless. She had previously been entirely well, having returned from a holiday to Australia two days previously. The day before admission she had noticed her left calf was a little swollen and had made an appointment to see her GP. The next day she collapsed in the street, acutely breathless. On examination in Casualty she was sweating and unwell with cold peripheries. Her respiratory rate was 50/min with a pulse of 130/min and blood pressure 85/40 mmHg. The venous pressure was raised to 15 cm above the sternal angle but the chest was completely clear. The left calf was red and swollen. Abdominal examination was unremarkable. An ECG showed sinus tachycardia, right axis deviation and right bundle branch block.

This patient is hypotensive with poorly perfused peripheries. A raised JVP in the absence of added heart sounds or lung crepitations suggests a 'pure' right-sided heart problem and in this case the likeliest cause is acute pulmonary embolism. The red swollen calf is in keeping with thrombosis of the deep veins of the legs, probably secondary to a period of prolonged immobilization on the flight from Australia.

AORTIC DISSECTION

This is a catastrophic condition caused by a tear in the intima of the aorta. Blood enters the wall of the aorta at high pressure and separates the middle and outer layers, creating a 'false lumen' filled with blood within the wall of the vessel. Occasionally it takes place in a normal aorta, but more frequently it arises in patients with longstanding hypertension. Another important association is with hereditary collagen diseases such as **Marfan's syndrome**.

The classical presentation of acute aortic dissection is with searing pain between the scapulae, often in association with central chest pain. Other presentations depend on the location of the intimal tear and its extension proximally or distally along the wall of the aorta. If blood tracks back to the aortic root, the architecture of the valvular ring is distorted. This leads to torrential AR which, because it happens so suddenly, is poorly tolerated and leads to left heart failure with pulmonary oedema. If the dissection involves the aortic arch the head and neck vessels may be involved leading to stroke. Renal and limb vessels may be similarly compromised if the dissection extends more distally.

The early treatment of aortic dissection involves diligent control of systolic blood pressure to 100 mmHg or less. Intravenous vasodilators such as sodium nitroprusside are most frequently used, often in combination with a β-blocker such as **propranolol**. It is not uncommon for several agents to be required to achieve good control. In descending aortic dissection surgery is generally not undertaken unless there are complications such as renal artery involvement. Proximal dissections require urgent CT scanning, transoesophageal echocardiography or aortography and surgical repair.

PRIMARY PULMONARY HYPERTENSION

In this condition a process of thickening and narrowing of the pulmonary arteries causes raised pressures in the pulmonary circulation with abnormally high resistance to right ventricular emptying. Most sufferers are young females and presentation is usually with breathlessness. Exertional syncope is another common symptom. With exercise peripheral resistance falls but systemic output cannot rise normally due to the limited amount of blood that the right ventricle can drive through the lungs into the left ventricle. Eventually right heart failure develops, with oedema and ascites, as a result of the chronically raised afterload placed on the right ventricle.

Examination shows a **parasternal heave** from an overworked right ventricle, oedema and a loud P_2 which may even be palpable.

Investigations show right ventricular hypertrophy on ECG and CXR.

Treatment is unsatisfactory. Calcium antagonists have been tried, as have continuous infusions of prostacyclin (a pulmonary vasodilator), but the prognosis is poor. Heart–lung transplantation is sometimes indicated.

CARDIOLOGICAL PROBLEMS IN PREGNANCY

During pregnancy cardiac output rises significantly in order to meet the requirements of the placenta. This is achieved through a rise in heart rate and an increase in preload as plasma volume expands during pregnancy. These extra demands placed on the heart may cause presentation of previously undiagnosed pathologies or exacerbate pre-existing cardiac defects.

The diagnosis of cardiac defects in pregnancy is made difficult by the fact that normal pregnancy may cause 'cardiac symptoms' of fatigue, exertional dyspnoea and ankle oedema. In addition, flow murmurs and added heart sounds are common due to the hyperdynamic circulation. The expanding uterus pushes on the diaphragm and may displace the cardiac apex laterally, producing axis changes on the ECG. Where there is diagnostic doubt echocardiography with Doppler studies identifies significant valvular abnormalities and seems to be safe to the fetus.

Pregnancy worsens the symptoms of **mitral stenosis** as the extra volume of blood in the vascular compartment cannot flow freely across the narrowed mitral valve. Life-threatening pulmonary oedema may occur, particularly during delivery, so treatment (where possible) should be with valvotomy before the onset of labour. Where this is not feasible careful supervision of diuretic therapy is required so as not to deplete the intravascular compartment too much, thereby threatening placental blood flow.

Prosthetic heart valves present a particular problem. Warfarin is associated with fetal abnormalities and is relatively contraindicated in the first trimester. It is important that women with prosthetic valves should plan their pregnancies carefully and many suggest that warfarin be stopped at the earliest opportunity and substituted with heparin for the first thirteen weeks. Warfarin may then safely be restarted but heparin is usually recommended towards term in case surgical intervention is required. Antibiotic prophylaxis against endocarditis is essential for all women with valvular disease undergoing any form of intervention during labour.

Hypertension may be pre-existing or develop in pregnancy. The commonest drugs used for treatment are α-methyl dopa and hydrallazine. **Pre-eclampsia** describes the association of hypertension, proteinuria and oedema and requires careful obstetric supervision as progression to **eclampsia** with cerebral oedema and convulsions carries a high mortality.

Pregnancy-associated cardiomyopathy

This seems to be a particular form of cardiomyopathy that develops towards the end of pregnancy, or just after. It is more common in multiparous women over the age of 30 and often presents with life-threatening pulmonary oedema. Early delivery is essential, after which cardiac function may improve. A higher morbidity and mortality is associated with each subsequent pregnancy.

Glossary of drugs in cardiology

Drug	Uses	Cautions/contraindications/side-effects
Amiloride	Heart failure Conservation of potassium with loop diuretics	Avoid in hyperkalaemia and renal failure May cause hyperkalaemia
Amiodarone	Commonly used in many ventricular and supraventricular arrhythmias	Sinus bradycardia, heart block thyroid dysfunction Side-effects include thyroid disturbance, lung fibrosis, corneal microdeposits, photosensitive rash, hepatitis
Amlodipine	Angina Hypertension	May cause or worsen hypotension
Aspirin	Acute MI, unstable angina and stable coronary disease	Occasionally precipitates bronchospasm May cause GI upset/bleeding
Atenolol	Angina Arrhythmias Hypertension	May worsen or precipitate heart failure, asthma, obstructive airways disease heart block, hypotension
Bendro-fluazide	Hypertension Heart failure	Avoid in renal failure May precipitate gout May cause hypokalaemia/hyponatraemia May cause or aggravate glucose intolerance
Bisoprolol	Angina Hypertension	May worsen or precipitate heart failure, asthma or obstructive airways disease heart block, hypotension

Bumetanide	Heart failure Oliguria due to renal failure	May cause hypokalaemia/hyponatraemia May precipitate gout May precipitate acute retention of urine (when used i.v.)
Captopril	Heart failure Hypertension	Avoid in aortic stenosis and renal failure May precipitate or worsen renal impairment May cause dry cough and hyperkalaemia
Digoxin	Heart failure Rate control in AF	Reduce dose in renal failure and in the elderly Avoid in AF with WPW
Diltiazem	Angina Hypertension Rate control in AF	May worsen or precipitate heart failure, hypotension, heart block
Disopyramide	AVNRT, AVRT Ventricular arrhythmias	Caution in heart failure, hypotension Avoid in heart block May cause dry mouth, urinary retention
Enalapril	Heart failure Hypertension	Avoid in aortic stenosis and renal failure May precipitate or worsen renal impairment May cause dry cough and hyperkalaemia
Flecainide	AVNRT, AVRT paroxysmal AF Ventricular arrhythmias	Avoid in heart failure Caution in coronary disease
Frumil (frusemide and amiloride)	Heart failure	May cause hyperkalaemia May precipitate gout
Frusemide	Heart failure Oliguria due to renal failure	May cause hypokalaemia/hyponatraemia May precipitate gout May precipitate acute retention of urine (when used i.v.) High doses may cause tinnitus and deafness

Glyceryl trinitrate (GTN)	Prophylaxis and relief of angina Breathlessness due to left ventricular failure	Often causes headache and flushing May cause dizziness and hypotension
Heparin	Anticoagulation in unstable angina Following tPA in acute MI DVT/PE	May cause haemorrhage May cause thrombocytopaemia and osteoporosis with prolonged usage
Isosorbide mononitrate	Prophylaxis of angina Heart failure	May cause headache, flushing, dizziness and hypotension
Lignocaine	Ventricular arrhythmias (especially following acute MI)	Reduce dose in heart failure, hepatic impairment Avoid in heart block, severe heart failure
Lisinopril	Heart failure Hypertension	Avoid in aortic stenosis and renal failure May precipitate or worsen renal impairment May cause dry cough and hyperkalaemia
Metoprolol	Angina Hypertension Arrhythmias	May worsen or precipitate heart failure, asthma or obstructive airways disease, heart block, hypotension
Mexiletine	Ventricular arrhythmias	Avoid in bradycardia, heart block
Nifedipine	Angina (with ß-blocker) Hypertension	May worsen or precipitate hypotension, heart failure
Propranolol	Angina Hypertension Arrhythmias	May worsen or precipitate heart failure, asthma or obstructive airways disease, heart block, hypotension
Ramipril	Heart failure Hypertension	Avoid in aortic stenosis and renal failure May precipitate or worsen renal impairment May cause dry cough and hyperkalaemia

Sotalol	Supraventricular and ventricular arrhythmias	May worsen or precipitate heart failure, asthma or obstructive airways disease heart block, hypotension
Spironolactone	Heart failure Oedema and ascites in liver cirrhosis Conservation of potassium with loop diuretics Hypertension due to Conn's syndrome	Avoid in hyperkalaemia and renal failure May cause gynaecomastia
Streptokinase	Acute MI Occasionally in massive PE	Avoid in recent stroke, active peptic ulceration, proliferative diabetic retinopathy, major surgery within previous 10 days or bleeding diathesis Caution if preceding prolonged and/or traumatic cardiac massage If streptokinase given more than 3 days previously then use tPA May cause bleeding, especially at intravenous puncture sites and intracerebrally
TPA (tissue plasminogen activator)	Acute MI	Avoid in recent stroke, active peptic ulceration, proliferative diabetic retinopathy, major surgery within previous 10 days or bleeding diathesis Caution if preceding prolonged and/or traumatic cardiac massage May cause bleeding, especially at intravenous puncture sites and intracerebrally
Verapamil	Angina Hypertension Rate control in AF AVNRT, AVRT	May worsen or precipitate heart failure, heart block, hypotension Avoid in AF with WPW
Warfarin	Prosthetic heart valves, AF, DVT, PE	Caution in hepatic disease Contraindicated in pregnancy May cause bleeding

Index

Page numbers appearing in **bold** refer to figures